I0474025

Dedicated to my wife for all
her love and patience...
Thank you

Table of Contents

Preface

It seems appropriate that this book is written after I have completed my Internal Medicine residency. I have finally had the chance to sit, gather my thoughts, and present them in some organized fashion so that it may have a profound and hopefully a lasting effect on my readers. As I browse the web, local bookstores, and now eBooks, it seems like every book written by physicians about health care is a collection of stories that aim to arouse emotion from their readers.

Certainly, our daily experiences make for fantastic stories that none can fabricate from scratch. Thus, it gives rise to television sitcoms that make millions off the drama of human life and "Life in the ER." As entertaining as these shows and books may be, none touch on the real challenges of today's health care. Moreover, young physicians are the least discussed. Shows like "Grey's Anatomy" cannot keep Hollywood out of the real stories. Such drama does not exist; where multiple relationships are taking place and social drama dominate daily work life. Nor is there a constant battle between the "janitor" and the resident where daily pranks are played out to see who wins at the end. Certainly, physicians are not so direct and clever on their feet where witty dialogues like from Dr. Cox can exist. There is no "barbie" on the wards, nor is there a depressed lawyer who randomly roams the halls with his singing choir.

All these sitcoms and movies create confusion to those who do not work in the health care field. Some may become motivated to emulate these Hollywood characters;

ultimately challenging the efficiency and effectiveness of the delivery of health care. In the mist of all this confusion, it is the patient who is at most risk.

So, the goal of this book is to fill this void. It is quite simple really. The focus is to share experiences through the eyes of a young resident who evolves into a more informed staff physician, while sharing stories as he matures and recognizes the challenges of health care least discussed. Life facilitates drama with the unavoidable clash between work and family. The dynamics of health care are changing at a rate where the profession is at real jeopardy. The aging population has provided the young generation with much energy, knowledge, and guidance, but yet we remain unprepared.

Change requires collaboration from physicians and non-physicians. Therefore, this book aims to inform the general public and give insight into the inner world of health care delivery. I hope to capture your attention into the emotions, critical decisions, and the issues that must be addressed to better prepare our future physicians. Program directors, administrators, mentors, and other health care personnel may also benefit in reading this book as health care is a complex institution composed of various individuals with various specialties who play critical roles in delivering health care. Thus, it is imperative that we understand this point – health care delivery must follow a team-based approach. The individualistic ideologies, the greed for fame and monetary reward, narcissistic behaviors, and the all preconceived opinions must be eradicated to effectively deliver health care.

Finally, upon completion of this book, the hope is that we can have a discussion on how to improve our medical education system, how to improve health care delivery in our academic hospitals, and how we as family members should work with health care personnel while our loved one is sick. Each one of us plays a role in the delivery of health care and these relationships must be recognized by all of us to assure proper and efficient patient care.

Moreover, young physicians must recognize these issues, educate themselves, and respond effectively. The older physicians must facilitate an environment where discussion, education, and empowerment can freely take place. It becomes quite apparent how dynamic and challenging health care is today. It is with this mindset we begin our discussion....

CHAPTER 1

Quiet Time

My feet were burning with pain and felt heavy as if I had walked a thousand miles across the country. I could tell they were swollen as my toes began to feel like they were running out of space in my Crocs. My white coat was heavy and hung over my shoulders like wet laundry on a string. My scrubs were wrinkled from what seemed to be an orchestra of movements consisting of sitting, standing, speed walking, and even running. My stethoscope hung around my neck causing a dull ache. I sat staring at a desktop computer that sat quietly in front of me. My eyes were exhausted from staring at labs and evaluating various radiology films; at times getting nose length away from the screen thinking that will help distinguish a spot I found on a film. The hallways had dim track lighting, which was usually done at night to help patients rest. The quiet halls were filled with distant sounds of tired nurses reminding each other of vitals and their daily assessments. The silence was pleasant, yet daunting in that one is uncertain what can happen at any minute. It is quite rare to have this peace, but when one finds himself/herself in this moment, we must make the most of it by closing our eyes, taking off our shoes, or simply reflect on life; which I tend to do.

I lifted my fatigued hands to the keyboard that lay in front of me and adjusted my glasses over my sweaty bridge of my nose only to slide further down my nose minutes later. I looked at my list of patients and started to follow up labs and assure proper documentation was completed on our electronic medical record system. Any resident will tell you that when we are doing this, we find ourselves having an internal dialogue and reminding ourselves of key components of each case. Thoughts race across your mind, eyes swing side to side navigating data quickly, and a story is formulated to possibly explain the abnormality. You create a mental image of the patient, followed by your physical exam. Then you find yourself thinking "what was the deal with that rash?" or "their labs look so good, why are they feeling miserable?" It is quite frequent that this explosion of interactions in the brain causes one to stop, close their eyes, and take a deep breath. This particular night, I needed to just stop and rest.

It was 3am. I had finally caught up with admitting seven patients, discussing with staff each case, discussing the case with on-call consultants, and "putting out fires," as we called it, on floor calls. In the mist of all this, there is a "rapid response" team that is composed of ICU nurses and the on-call senior resident, who attend to patients that are not doing well and may have a change in clinical status requiring urgent attention. These moments call for rapid communication and decision making, involving the patient, nursing staff, and other physicians who either are involved in the case already or need to be invited to join the case. Undoubtedly, there are a few of these a night which adds to the chaos of these night calls.

I was a third year Internal Medicine resident on night call in my final months, where I found myself simply exhausted and full of reflection. In a single night, I had managed acute seizure, severe pneumonia, blood infections, kidney failure, vomiting blood, to heart failure where their lungs are full of fluid causing them to have trouble breathing. I smiled at the thought of this because it is truly amazing the amount of data you process, decisions you make, and the interactions you have that no matter how you tell your story about your night, none can truly experience it as you had. In looking at my computer and the electronic record, I began to think of how different medicine is today. It is incredible how medicine has changed and how I was part of this change. On this night, I had to ask myself, is the change for the better or worse? Moreover, are people aware of these changes and how they affect young physicians?

CHAPTER 2

Humiliation

It was 5am when my alarm went off with "What is Love" (Baby Don't Hurt Me, No More) by Haddaway, which I must admit put a smile on my face. I turned only to find my wife sound asleep in her usual curled up in a ball position. I kissed her on the cheek, which usually elicited a "emmm, what time is it?" in a tired and cracking voice. To this I usually replied, "game time."

Every morning was the same; very monotonous and predictable. It usually started with the stumble to the bathroom with half shut eyes, trying to find my way to the bathroom in a dark room; tip-toeing and evading roadside barriers that are left on the floor from the previous chaotic day. Once in the bathroom, you had the brushing of teeth, shower, shirt, tie, and then breakfast that had to include a nice tall coffee to go. My wife usually met me by the kitchen with a big smile and lunch packed in an old grocery bag (I used to have a lunch bag but lost it on one of my rotations and buying another was another expense that we had to think twice about).

The drive to the hospital usually involved listening to NPR and a time for reflection. I usually thought about the previous day and what I had missed or what I had to improve on. On one particular morning, I was thinking about how residents are treated in the hospital.

It seems as though the old perception of residents as "work horses" has still not left the minds of most individuals. Moreover, it is not foreign to any resident when certain staff members in the hospital make comments like, "well, I make way more than you and you have to do almost five times the work I do." My personal favorite is "are you sure you want to complete this residency?" And most of us have heard the all too familiar "So, when you graduate don't you have like hundreds of thousands of dollars in student loans to payback? Wow, I would never be a doctor!"

What is interesting about all this is that when one enters their first year of residency, we expect it. We expect disrespect, the constant sarcastic humiliation from staff members, and the long sleepless nights. But, as one matures and becomes more informed, confident in the delivery of medicine, such practices are extremely distasteful. Being an intern in any residency program demands patience and the ability to stay quiet when others humiliate you. Is this the proper culture to begin medical training? Think about it for a second. You have an individual who has been working hard at maintaining their grade point average since high school, studying hard to score in the upper percentile of all standardized testing through college and finally though medical school only to be humiliated and disrespected the minute they earn the title of a medical resident. How can we tolerate such a culture? Moreover, it begs the question whether such treatment happens only in the United States? The respect for physicians, especially young physicians is at an all time low. But who is to blame? How did we get here?

I remember one particular busy afternoon where a nurse had asked me about what do with her patient who's Port-a-cath (permanent centeral catheter placed under skin usually in cancer patient to prevent frequent needle sticks for access) was not drawing blood. I was an intern at the time and did not know the best solution to the problem. So, I asked what she has tried and what our options are in this situation. To this, she quickly snapped, "You have no idea what a port-a-cath is, do you?" With a disgusted face she abruptly turned around and left while I was in mid sentence trying to discuss potential solutions. Staring at an empty wall, I was floored at how I was treated and looked around if anyone had witnessed this interaction. One nurse was slamming away on a keyboard as she was finishing her progress note and looked up with a smirk as if to say, "sucks to be you."

Every resident can also recall busy nights where you are working on admissions as fast as you can and are called by a nurse whose only words are, "yeah, we just received a transfer and I need orders." There has been a movement towards limiting verbal orders, which makes this interaction most difficult. There is no way one can be at two places at once. What ends up happening is the resident would say that they are in the ER and will come as soon as possible. At times, this interaction is smooth when the nurse and resident work as a team. Verbal orders can be given and basic labs can be drawn in the meantime to facilitate the admission process. Other times, there is this terrible interaction where the conversation can end up with the nurse hanging up on the resident who is in mid sentence.

I remember when I was at the VA (Veterans Affairs) Medical Center where I was disputing with a nurse regarding a blood pressure that was mildly elevated in an asymptomatic patient. She insisted that I give some medication to lower it, but I reminded her that this is not in the best interest of the patient. This discussion became hostile and she ended up hanging up on me. This was not the first time I was treated this way, so it does not affect you much. But we have to ask, is any young professional suppose to be treated this way? Moreover, does this not bring tension in the management team who is taking care of the patient, which ultimately may jeopardize the health of the patient?

These experiences definitely affect the development of any professional. Some may take these experiences from the "I survived it so everyone else has to" perspective. Others may take this as an opportunity for change and will make a personal mission not to treat their residents and students this way. Personally, I did not handle these criticisms well initially. It was a culture shock. I had gone from being the cream of the crop with academics to total humiliation. The smiles of approval and acceptance abruptly halted and were quickly replaced with harsh criticism. Each day was a challenge. I woke up asking myself, "why am I doing this again?" I remember having a conversation with friends and family who have graduated from college, had small businesses, or were in graduate school, but nonetheless did not have the humongous debt over their head nor this constant battle with disrespect on a daily basis. How is this motivating or fair?

The fact of the matter is that medical student and resident behavior have been studied for years. Moreover, it has become clear that in any demanding and stressful occupations, like health care, depression and anxiety are quite common. Fatigue and burnout are equally common threats to the profession. However, what are residency programs doing to prevent burnout? Are there solutions in place to deal with resident burnout? We lack prospective trials that show beneficial solutions in preventing and treating resident burnout. Depression, anxiety, and lack of job satisfaction are real threats to an already troubled health care system. This issue of emotional/physical fatigue, burnout, depression, and anxiety are not issues of just the American student. It is present in health care professionals across the world! So, we obviously do not have control of the situation.

In the first six months of my intern year I seriously questioned my career path. Fortunately I had my masters in health care administration, so the thought of giving up and utilizing those skills were constantly entertained. But, that was not the plan! The goal was to be a well informed physician from a medical and business standpoint so I can effectively make changes to this already flawed system. It was a hill that seemed endless.

I remember being in ICU rounds, presenting a complicated patient to the ICU team and was interrupted by the pulmonary fellow who said, "actually we did not do that this morning, we actually changed our minds." Really!! If this is my patient, why was I not informed! The anger was too much for me to bear. This was a common practice where the interns are simply reporting what the fellow and the senior resident who is supervising them did that morning. Why don't I just go back to wearing that small medical student jacket instead of this long over-filled, dirty, worthless lab coat!

It is this very moment that I had an epiphany. Every man is for himself. Medicine was my business and the reality is, no one on that team or any future team truly cared for my business or my success. The only way I could change that culture was not by yelling, screaming, or even showing my anger. Besides, I was just a resident. Even worse, I was an intern. So, I had to remain silent, internalize these emotions, and wait for my turn to change the system. As time passed, I knew I had to work from the ground up. Gain the credibility of the nursing staff, gain their trust, and ultimately gain the respect my attending. This would take time and effort. It is this realization that changed me forever.

CHAPTER 3

Rounding Charades

I arrived at the hospital several minutes early to my usual time. The parking lot was usually empty with a few cars that sat in the quiet early morning hours. The brisk morning air was cool to the face. I gathered my bag from the back seat and started the usual dreaded walk to the front entrance. Few other people joined me in this quiet walk; all looking fatigued from the prior day and looking at the ground as they somehow navigated their way to the front door. Why is it that we always look at the floor while we walk? It's as if we are so tired that we can't even lift our head up when we walk. The amazing truth is that we seem to be able to navigate our way with our head down. Truly amazing!

Once inside the hospital, the bright lights and the unnecessary décor always seem to wake me up. It is truly fascinating the significant investment hospitals make in decorating their front entrance. Our hospital had glass artwork hanging from the ceilings with modern furniture providing seating for an overpriced café that sat in the corner. Large windows bordered the front entrance so people from the outside can see these luxurious accommodations. I guess this brings comfort to visitors as they enter the hospital and possibly create the illusion of entering a facility that is at the "cutting edge" of medicine.

The "ding" of the elevator always brought more sadness as it reminded me that work was getting closer. The chaos that existed on the wards was near. It truly seems like you are entering a time warp or some tunnel as you go up this elevator to the wards. Once you are on the floor, time seems to accelerate and all of a sudden time becomes your enemy. People recognize your arrival and are not shy to come up to you for some verbal orders before you even get settled. At times, emergencies catch you off guard and you literally have to drop your bag at the nursing station and help with the emergency. So, the elevator is your last stop before you enter the chaos.

Once off the elevator, I walked to my team room, maximizing the enjoyment of my freedom with each step. Thankfully, on this particular day, there were no emergencies. I was able to walk to my team room without any pit stops. Once inside my team room, I was surrounded by the sound of interns pounding away on their keyboards; navigating, reading, and learning their patients on their list quickly as possible. As a supervising second year resident, the job is to coordinate a team to assure proper care is delivered. It is a very responsible position, but the role can vary depending on the staff. At times, you are treated as a colleague or teammate with the staff, but other times, you are part of the "scut" team. Once the morning rounds were done by us – "the scut team"- it was time for academic rounds.

Academic rounds are quite entertaining if you think about it. You have the attending staff member who is usually several years older than the rest of the team members who is followed by a long train of individuals. Nowadays, there are the COWS (computers on wheels) which are truly dangerous when you have medical students who are busy working on their notes while driving these dangerous vehicles. We actually had a staff member who was "run over" by one of these and it was not pretty. The staff physician was one of the most respected, most hard working, and most intense physician in the history of the hospital and when his face turns red, we all duck for cover; which is exactly what happened.

The staff physician is followed by tired residents whose coats are full of papers, books, food stains at times, and reviewing their patient presentation in their head as they near the patient they are taking care of. The medical students are always at the end of this train, usually walking just as fast and nervous about their presentations. Finally, there are the pharmacists, social worker, and case manager at times that complete this train of people. Making a patient presentation requires the medical student to first step in front and present in an organized manner. They usually are surrounded by the rest of the team, some who are pounding away on their laptop working on notes, others step aside to answer pages, others look through their pagers, and finally there are those who just stare at the students to intimidate them. As the student starts their presentation, the staff usually has the look of "I wonder what game is on tonight?" or "Boy, I am pretty tired today. I gotta round faster." The student goes through the overnight events, physical exam, and then assessment and plan. Once the presentation is completed, then start the repeated questions from the staff, which only screams "I wasn't listening, but I am going to ask you to repeat yourself one more time, simply because I am a staff physician!" This is followed by rhetorical questions from the staff physician who plays a game called "Everyone, guess what I am thinking!" This can go on for some time, which delays the morning rounds.

Teaching rounds should be concise, efficient, and timely. Each patient presentation should be respected. Nurses do join these presentations and play critical roles in decision-making. However, here is where the problem lies.

So, the medical student presents a particular patient that he/she is following, and there is usually an intern that follows that patient as well. The senior resident also is aware of the patient as he/she is responsible for the entire service. I guarantee every resident in the United States has been in a situation where either you are presenting or a medical student is, but the senior resident or the nurse says, "Actually, we did not do that today, we did this instead." It makes the student and intern feel less important and not part of the team. I used to have the hardest time as an intern to get help from the nursing staff. They are usually busy completing their assessments, checking out to other nurses, or simply tired and the last thing they want to do is talk to an intern about a patient. But, this not only left me frustrated and angry because this would lead to inconsistent and incomplete presentations, but the feeling of not being part of the treatment team could not be ignored. This leads to disinterest, distrust, and not enjoying patient care.

During the rounds of questioning and teaching, at times I felt these were not fair. Some residents are ridiculed for their lack of knowledge and the inability to answer promptly when asked for quick recall. Ridicule has a profound effect on the treatment team. Again, rounds are attended by not just physicians, but other health personnel. Thus, ridicule threatens the credibility of team members. For example, when an intern is ridiculed in rounds, he/she may come around to check on a patient and may order certain things only to be questioned by the nursing staff. This may delay the delivery of care and leave the resident feeling distrusted. It is quite amazing how fast rumors and stories pass around the hospital as well. Each resident is constantly being evaluated by people they may know and even not know. Therefore, it is imperative that young physicians realize that their effectiveness is determined by the trust they gain from their health care team. This means, they must monitor how they behave, what they say, and how they treat everyone in the hospital. One's demeanor certainly can set the tone of the treatment team. Hollywood taints this and urges physicians to be "cool" and "relaxed." There are limits to this; however, it must be stressed that full embracement of such behavior comes with a bag full of risks. One must wonder if the changing personality of physicians has led to some of the lack of respect or mistreatment of physicians today.

It may not be a horrible idea for team building exercises to be done at an organizational level including the residents and students. Hospitals are huge organizations with multiple players. Thus, it is reasonable to think that a team building exercise with the treatment team (physicians, nurses, residents, and students) can improve their delivery of health care. Why not? The product they are manufacturing together is service. The physician – nurse dynamic has been discussed for some time now. But why is it not implemented across the country? Is it because of a clash between the aging physicians and new ideas? The team approach to patient care and rounding starts with the physician-nurse dynamic. This interaction is so important that it will set the tone for the rest of the treatment team members. More importantly, it will demonstrate unity and uniformity in the delivery of patient care.

Why is it that we apply business tools and practice methods to hospitals when it comes to finances, but completely fail in applying human resources, marketing, and most importantly organizational communication to the health care setting?

CHAPTER 4

Something Called Communication

Most physicians who have been in practice for some time will agree that the respect for physicians has diminished over the years. Who is to blame? On one hand, you have the interactions with nurses who are governed by policies and strive on a daily basis to assure they follow "protocol" to protect their jobs. However, on the other hand, you have physicians who are trying to reduce their liability and are trying to see as many patients as they can to satisfy the needs of administration. All this is done under a stressful environment where a patients' life awaits the decisions that come from all these interactions. Thus, it feeds a complex situation.

Documentation at times becomes the only means of communication between health care professionals. To some, it may seem surprising that there are still hospitals that operate with hand written notes. There is an enormous push for a complete electronic record. This change will take several years. Either way, in a busy hospital, these notes become the only means of communication. Unfortunately, the biggest challenge is getting the physician and nurse to round together. Why is that? Why is this simple principle not aggressively pursued or implemented? Is the value of revenue greater than the quality of patient care?

Did you ever try reading a physician handwritten note? It is like unscrambling an ancient scroll! In all seriousness, if these hand written notes are a significant means of communicating between health care professionals, why is are they so illegible? Furthermore, if any administrator were to realize how inefficient care is when people cannot read or understand what is written, then investing in a complete electronic medical record is obvious. In addition to poorly written notes, the sacred time for performing a physical exam is becoming compromised.

There are times during the physical exam or when a physician enters a patient's room, a nurse will be in the background adjusting, starting, changing various drips, all which produce noise and clouds the interaction with the patient. As a resident, I remember being interrupted constantly. It seemed as though the nurses would wait until I would walk into the room so they can interrupt me the moment I opened my mouth. Any resident can attest that most of these questions were so senseless that it made one wonder what exactly made the matter so urgent.

Nonetheless, it was expected that you pause turn to the nurse and answer their nonsense question; all with a great big smile and a "sure, no problem". It's not like residents are under significant time restraints to see more than ten sick patients with multiple organ failure, while researching a treatment plan to present on rounds so they don't embarrass themselves. Never mind the pager that constantly beeps like an annoying child sitting in the back seat yelling, "are we there yet?!"

What happen to the moments where a physician can close the door behind him/her and have that uninterrupted sacred time with the patient? Has medicine changed so much that we need to be moving faster and do not have time for this patient-physician interaction? Have physicians been too lenient on this and allowed their physical exam time to be disturbed or are physicians themselves becoming less proficient with their physical exam skills with the advent of technology that the importance of this sacred time is lost? Finally, is it the fact that hospitals are run on efficiency so this time is automatically rushed and so there is no time to waste; speed overcomes actual efficiency given the significant amount of information or data that is missed given the lack of time with a patient?

Therefore, communication is vital in the health care setting. I would argue it is more important in this setting than in any other setting. Patients, nurses, family members, and the entire treatment team that includes pharmacy and social services must understand and respect the value of communication. The sense of a medical team is being lost. A team based approach to patient care is extremely important now more than ever. Thus, communication between team members is critical to assure each member understands their specific role in delivering patient care. We must approach patient care as a system where multiple players are involved. Each member offers unique skills and knowledge to each case. The physician is the leader of this team and has the ultimate responsibility of utilizing these skills most efficiently; providing the best care possible. For example, interdisciplinary rounds have shown some benefit in improving communication. This is where the physician, nurse, case manager, social worker, and pharmacist all sit down and discusses a case. It is an opportunity to get everybody together and gain insight from each member about a case. However, the challenge is finding this time. Again, hospital beds continue to rise without a consideration for appropriate staffing. Moreover, how often do we find large meeting rooms on hospital wards? As hospitals continue to expand and build fancier wards, why are there not many "team rooms?" The incentives and priorities are not in the right place. We have to go back to the basics where we find a way to allow all team members to come together and more importantly round together. If this is not possible, as physicians, we must find ways to efficiently lead our treatment teams. Certainly, at the end of the day, it is the physician that is ultimately in charge of a patients' care; no one else. Thus, it is not administration that cures a patient; rather, it is the physician.

In our litigious society, people are protecting themselves and are quick to say "I did my part." It is as if there are these imaginary check lists that we are expected to do. If one forgets to complete or check a particular box, then that person might as well kill somebody. The amount of emails, protocol violations, and the number of people that will start talking is ridiculous. It seems people who you always wondered what they do in the hospital all of a sudden have jobs and are quick to point out what should have been done. This leads to the long winded and unnecessary meetings where people come together to hear themselves talk, but no decisions are actually made.

We must work as a team to provide the most efficient and effective health care to our patients. This includes resident physicians. What kind of message are we sending to these young physicians? These interactions are not unique to any single hospital; one can find this across the country. But it is these interactions that tarnish the relationships between doctors and nurses, or other members of the medical team. Physicians are leaders of the medical team and any lawsuit tends to remind us of that which seems to be lost. Everyone is aware of the stories where in teaching rounds the nurse or some part of the medical team does not agree with the plan of care. This should launch an intellectual discussion between the members. Instead of hostility, people should share their knowledge. There are several times where the art of medicine comes into play. The physician may know of a particular treatment plan which tends to work whose scientific reason may not be hundred percent accurate. Nonetheless, we must try it to see if the patient improves. Medicine is very scientific, but we forget that it is an art as well. At the end of the day, we are human beings treating human beings. Thus, there are innate limitations to the practice of medicine. We all forget our natural mortality and even physicians who are reminded on a daily basis tend to forget theirs as well.

One solution that seems to work from personal experience is to get a hold of the nurse during rounds. In addition, having the nurse join you in the discussion with the family and the patient is very helpful. We must teach this method to our residents. We must teach them the importance of communication on rounds and leading a team of health care professionals. Having the social worker during rounds also helps. When the physician, nurse, and the social worker all enter the room together, it has a profound effect on the patient. First and foremost it demonstrates unity in the delivery of care. It easily becomes apparent that everyone is on the same page and talking to one another. There is nothing more frustrating for a patient than receiving conflicting information from their health care providers. Secondly, it is a more efficient visit. Several questions can be answered and decisions can be made together. Thus, the practice of medicine demands team work and communication that facilitates a team approach to patient care. One of the large barriers to communication is the "personality salad" at every hospital.

CHAPTER 5

Can You Come Talk To the Family...

It is not uncommon to find various personalities throughout the hospital, but it seems as though as the hospital gets busier, the ugliness consumes the entire hospital, which usually happens at night – as all evil does. As a senior resident on call, I was responsible for admitting patients, helping my interns with floor calls, running a code blue, and being part of the rapid response team. My night usually started at 7pm where I would get a checkout from the short call senior resident. This is a brief synopsis of the admissions he/she has done from 4pm to 7pm. It is also when any new admissions or the patients that are in the ER who need to be admitted are discussed. The interns at this same time are getting check out from various medicine teams regarding floor patients to the night call intern. So for example, each of the two interns on call has about three to four services to cover and each service has close to sixteen patients. So do the math. When called at night regarding any of these patients, the intern has to learn the patient quickly, understand the issue at hand, and then make recommendations with documentation. Each intern is provided a "check out" sheet. This sheet has a list of patients for each service with rows of information categorized from basic demographics to issues and management goals.

Let's look at this more closely here. So, when an intern gets called at 8pm regarding a patient, which usually involves a request by a nurse "to talk to the family." This is the most idiotic phenomenon that is happening in most academic centers. Why should an intern, whose only understanding of the patient is off of a sheet of paper and even when they do the best investigation of the patient as possible, they do not have much to offer to the family at 8pm. So here is what usually happens that leads to frustrated families. The intern will quickly read the sheet they have, recall the checkout they had received, and they go to the bedside and open the electronic record to investigate more regarding the patient. Prepared with basic information they would enter the patients' room. As most occasions, the family is sitting at the bedside with various expressions. There are those family members who will give you the nod of acknowledgement, those that smile – usually the grandmothers do this, and then you have the ones who glare at you as if you have just been convicted of a heinous crime and are awaiting the electric chair. Then, the questions begin. Almost always, they come all at once. As a resident, you answer to the best of your ability and say things like, "yes, the primary team will address that in the morning" or "I am only the covering resident at night and am unaware of any further plans at this time." The latter is what sets off the usual comments that include "Don't you know? Why do you not know? Don't you guys all talk."

To expand on this further, one must understand the complexity of today's patient. The patient today is becoming more complex with social challenges that continuously become even more difficult. The aging population, poor access to health care, and the poor economy all challenge the present delivery of health care. Thus, more specialists are involved in a patients' care now than ever before. Moreover, as a society, we tend to demand to see a "specialist" even for the most minor illness. This just feeds the rising cost of health care.

Nonetheless, as more specialists are involved the more complex the case gets not only in treating the pathology, but also coordination of care. Physicians have different personalities too. You have those who think they are God's gift to the world and then you have those who are humble and strive to do the best. As an internist or a primary caretaker of the patient, one must be able to "manage" these various personalities. Thus, once again, communication becomes vital in assuring the specialists and the rest of the treatment team is consistent in their patient care. Medical students and residents must learn how to lead their fellow physicians. Whether you are a surgeon, internist, family physician, gynecologist, or any physician, you will at some point be the primary caretaker of a patient.

Leadership and communication skills are lacking in our present day physicians. Administration can help facilitate this by allowing them to lead at an executive level. Meanwhile, physicians who are in leadership must educate the young generation towards strengthening their leadership skills. Personal growth requires not only obtaining knowledge but also a supportive environment where growth is demanded. Health care today is challenging as more people have multiple comorbidities with poor access to health care. The human body is unique in that each individual is different and no matter how much we try to generalize, there will always be a case that will surprise us.

Little do people understand that during each call night, a physician is looking after several patients. Each patient comes with not just one problem, but one problem that has affected multiple systems. Questions or events that do not require urgent attention must wait for the morning. It is impossible for families to expect 24hr service that is just as thorough as morning rounds. Quite frankly, people want their physicians to stand ready at minutes' notice.

Even more bothersome, people expect the same physician to respond at all times. Physicians are human beings too; with families, and the need for food and rest. Furthermore, clinical status of any patient can change so frequently that it is impossible to provide any guarantee to any management plan. What is interesting is that we tend to forget that we are all human beings and as much as we like to think we have control of the human body – we really don't.

CHAPTER 6

What Does It Mean To Be
A Physician?

Physicians do the best we can to improve quality of life and increase survival. That is it. The end result of all human life is death whether we like it or not. It is that simple. All of the research that we do focuses on improving survival and quality of life. Regardless, nothing will change the fact that we all will die at one point. Furthermore, the human body is so complex that pathologies occur that we conveniently call "idiopathic." This means, "I have no idea." For some reason there are gene mutations, some chemical interaction, or some infection decides to reactivate at a single particular moment for an unknown reason. These are factors that no human being can change. In having said that, one cannot ignore the humility and humbleness one feels. In a sense all humanity is united by this single fate. Therefore, it follows then why do we make it so difficult to have access to health care, or have uncontrolled rising cost of health care, and the aggressive pursuit for negligent physicians?

As a young resident physician, you are only introduced to the sickness of our own health care system. Medical school does not prepare their students regarding the inequalities, the barriers in accessing health care, or address the rising cost of health care. Never mind the lack of education regarding health law, interpersonal communication, or finance. Even if such courses are offered, they are taught at the end of the second year when each medical student could care less and is anxiously awaiting their third year rotations. We are trained solely to identify the pathological illness and treat it. Quite honestly, isn't that what the American people demanded of physicians until recently when this ugly monster became out of control? Physicians were never politicians and were never involved in the policy-making process. We have well-informed politicians with law backgrounds making decisions on how patient care should be done and statisticians with no health care training working in Medicare trying to figure out how much each diagnosis or procedure should cost. Now you have a situation where a young physician who probably wanted to become a physician solely for the reward of helping people when they are in their most vulnerable state, exposed to questions and personalities that only leave a sick feeling in ones stomach.

At times, I found myself questioning what it truly meant to be a physician. Am I demanded to simply diagnose and treat, or am I suppose to be more than that? If I am demanded to do more than that, then why was I not trained to do so? Is this supposed to be a great surprise!

The present day physician is not required to just diagnose and treat an illness. Physicians are demanded to implement treatment plans by leading a team of other physicians, nurses, techs, pharmacists, social work, case managers, and other ancillary staff. Leading a team towards treating a patient requires communication and management skills to maintain motivation and focus. Once the patient is better, the discharge plan must be coordinated and resources like home health, home physical therapy, nursing home, skilled nursing facility, and financial assistance for medications must exist. It is the physician that becomes the voice, the representative of the patient to assure these resources are aligned for a safe discharge. It becomes apparent that the physician becomes not only a leader of patient care inside the hospital, but is actively involved with government programs, insurance companies, pharmaceutical industry, and long term care facilities that exist outside the hospital. The physician is at the center of a massive web of entities that demand their leadership. So, are our young physicians prepared for this task?

I was raised watching my moms' family practice flourish with patients satisfied and thankful for her care. I witnessed the transformation of patient care from a paternal relationship to a more mutual relationship between patient and physician. The advent of the World Wide Web allowed patients to become informed, but also flooded them with misinformation. Thus, it gave rise to confusion and distrust. Family members were becoming more aggressive and the interaction between the physician and family became stressful situations and at times hostile. I notice this especially when the physician is from another country. The accent itself becomes a challenge and I feel as much as our medical schools do a poor job in teaching communication, foreign graduates who are not originally born in America are at an even more of a disadvantage.

So, it is important for all of us understand the importance of these interactions. Moreover, as family members, we must be patient. How can one effectively simplify the complex processes and physiological interactions that are at play in an ill patient? Moreover, how can one demonstrate the severity of an illness while balancing the emotions of the patient and their families? As physicians, we are constantly watching the families' reaction as we begin to explain the illness. We constantly ask ourselves, how can I explain this critical or terminal illness in the most simple, empathic, and less devastating way? It is not a simple task. All this is done while keeping our composure, controlling our own emotions; as we must demonstrate strength and be ready to provide support to loved ones.

So you see, when it comes to the interaction between physicians and family members, both are involved in an incredible mental exercise. You have the family members eager to get their questions answered, trying to remember all they wanted to ask before the physician escapes from their site. Then you have the physician who is processing information, thinking out loud at times, and formulating the best delivery of all the information that needs to be communicated in the most effective way. Never mind the constant interruptions of cell phones, pagers, nurses calling out, or beeps of pumps and monitors that may be in the room.

We must have mutual respect when it comes to this interaction. Physicians must realize the importance of the patients' family in patient care and the family must recognize and respect the physicians' effort in communicating this information effectively. The biggest investment in patient care a physician can make is the time that is spent with the family. But, where are the incentives to encourage such behavior?

In a time where physicians have so many patients to see whether it is in the clinic or in the hospital, time becomes our nemesis. Each interaction has an imaginary stopwatch above it running continuously until the physician rushes out the door. The nurse to patient ratio is so stretched that each nurse cannot possibly be expected to know everything about their patient. They have to scale it down to the basics: why were they admitted, what are we doing for them, and what is the discharge plan. Let's not forget the documentation that needs to support these interactions. So, if these interactions are not documented, then those interactions essentially did not happen and cannot be billed based on time.

Finally, are we training our young residents to appreciate and respect these family interactions? We do a great job hooking up cameras to see how they interact with patient actors in a controlled setting. But when they are on the wards, how many physicians take the time to see how the medical student and resident explain pathophysiology to family members? There simply is no time, nor is there enough of an incentive to do that.

A potential solution for all this is for the family to write down a list of questions prior to meeting with the physician. If the list is long and may take up more time, they can simply hand the list to the nurse who can help with most of their questions. If we had more nurses on the wards and physicians and nurses worked as a team, then communicating with family members is quite easy. Patient care is more efficient and leads to better patient satisfaction.

Our incentives in this country are not in the right place when it comes to health care. Hospitals must realize that it is critical to invest in patient satisfaction, family satisfaction, and basics of customer service. Almost all corporations realize this, why don't hospitals? Oh, that's right, when people are sick, their insurance or the government will pay! Not necessarily. In this day and age, patients will and should shop for the best hospitals and physicians who will manage their care to their personal satisfaction. It is more cost effective to invest in customer service by empowering medical staff to make decisions together, work as a team, and provide the medical staff with resources to provide the most efficient care.

CHAPTER 7

The Primary Caretakers

In my experience, I have realized family members are the primary care takers of any patient. The sad cases are those patients who have no families, or have broken relationships with their families. It is reasonable to be concerned about the medical care of a family member. It is the responsibility of the medical staff to effectively communicate the medical treatment to family members. Once a patient is admitted to the hospital, a medical team is launched and takes charge of treating that patient. Moreover, the primary physician is the leader in inviting specialists to the case if needed. However, most of the time, we forget the family members in this picture or the family members are timid and are unclear as to their role. I argue that family members become part of the team at the time of admission and should play an important role through the hospitalization up to the discharge of a patient. It is imperative that the value of family-physician communication be stressed just as much as patient-physician communication. If we fail to recognize this void, then the entire medical team suffers including the patient.

The fact of the matter is that the medical team can spend thousands of dollars and make a patient better, but it makes no sense to discharge a patient with no education and more importantly not educating their primary care takers. This recognition is a major player in reducing repeat hospitalizations for the same issue. In our busy hospitals we find the discharge day to be like a pit stop. The nurses, students, and physicians all go over the medications quickly and leave the patient with a handful of papers that don't make sense when they go home. This begins the cycle of not being followed up in clinic and the patient returns to the hospital sick again. In the meantime, the family becomes frustrated over all the paper work and the repeated hospitalization. Ultimately, this inefficiency significantly raises the cost of health care.

One of the most rewarding experiences I had was when I went over the medication list and appointments with a patient at the bedside. The act of just sitting down next to the patient can do volumes for creating a sense of comfort. I had called the son using her bedside phone and went over the list of medications and appointments. This simple act, which honestly took fifteen minutes, was much appreciated by the son who is the patient's primary care taker. Now having said this, I also noticed how cruel our health care system can be to some of our patients who cannot afford medications.

Every resident in the United States can attest to taking care of a patient with pulmonary disease and having the most difficult time getting inhalers at discharge for a patient who does not have insurance and cannot afford to pay for them without insurance. It makes no sense. I remember being on the phone with pharmacy for over an hour in trying to come up with creative ideas to get inhalers to a patient who needed them desperately. Our social worker was calling companies and searching for any assistance programs that may help in getting this patient his inhalers. All this discussion over a single patient, with a list of other patients to discharge when you are a resident becomes extremely overwhelming and frustrating.

Especially on discharge day, dealing with issues such as this delays the discharge. Even worse is when the resident finally makes it to the next patient, he/she is met with glaring eyes and disgust. Nurses may help the situation, but usually the family members are told "well, the doctor didn't sign the orders yet?" No matter how long you sit and tell family members regarding the previous patient and the difficult time you are having in getting the patient to afford inhalers that are life saving, you are asked a single question " so, did you sign the orders yet?"

It makes no sense to increasing access to health care and not addressing this issue of rising cost of prescription medicine. Simple inhalers that are life saving are so inflated that we are literally killing our own people for personal gain. How does this sit well with pharmaceutical companies? I felt terrible discharging my patient with pulmonary disease with one month supply of inhalers because that was the best we could do. Even then, when I walked in to shake his hand and give him his prescriptions, he said in a raspy voice "Doc, you have no idea how much I appreciate this. Thank you." I could only nod because I knew if I had said anything more or stayed in that room any longer the tears that were welling up in my eyes would pour down my face. I left the room saying to myself "this just isn't fair!"

Has capitalism become this monster that now governs our morality? If we realize the fact that we all will face the same end to our lives, how can we turn away from this issue? How can medicine be so expensive? How can other countries offer medicine at cheaper prices? As the most powerful nation on this planet how are we not taking care of our own people? Unfortunately, people are choosing unhealthy lifestyles these days and come to our ER's to get care, only not to pay for the services rendered –

which only adds to the rising cost of health care. It's a problem that we all are at fault.

Over time, it becomes apparent, that no matter how much we take care of ourselves certain patients who are immunosuppressed or have a number of comorbidites, which unfortunately is not hard to find these days, will be hospitalized several times. It is at those moments, where a patient is having multiple hospitalizations with the same issue or it becomes evident that the patient is getting worse, it calls for active participation between family members, the patient, and the medical team.

CHAPTER 8

Still Full Code...

The most horrific experience any physician can have is the one where the family decides to continue aggressive medical treatment in a patient who has a terminal illness. Just as a side, this concept of "terminal illness" is hilarious because isn't any illness going to at some point wear down our system to a point where eventually our body will begin to accumulate irreversible damage?

We had a patient who had metastatic lung cancer was more than eighty years old and had been admitted with pneumonia that was so significant that his kidneys, heart, and brain were affected. It was documented and discussed with family members on numerous occasions the aggressive nature of the cancer and this pneumonia that seemed to have a devastating impact on the human body. I remember being on teaching rounds and standing behind my staff while he explained to them the aggressiveness of the pneumonia and that the patient had been requiring more oxygen in the last twenty-four hours and was on eight liters of nasal cannula (the oxygen device that fits under the nose). We explained that this pneumonia had lead to an infection in the blood and the systems were showing signs of shutting down. With this came the discussion of code status. For some reason, people associate this discussion as "throwing in the towel." The patient by this point was delirious and was not participating in the conversation, his DPOA (Durable Power of Attorney) was his wife, and of course he did not have a living will. So, the decision-making was left to his wife.

Now to put this situation in perspective, you have a room filled with the staff physician at the bedside looking over the patient who is mostly sleepy, about three residents behind the staff probably shifting their weight between each leg to reduce the pain, a nurse case manager, a pharmacist, about three medical students in their short white coat jackets with eyes tearing at the sight of a dying patient, and finally a social worker also wearing a white coat. On the other side of the bed are the family members who are usually about 7-10 in number. The wife is usually sitting, nervous at the idea of being in charge of making further decisions. The other family members are standing surrounding the wife. The room is usually quiet and begins to feel warm given all the people in this single room.

"Now, one of the things we have to decide is if the patient will like to proceed with life saving measures" says my staff.

This usually triggers several emotions in the room. Some people start to cry, others begin to look down at their feet, and there are other family members who will become angry at the mention of "life saving." At this particular instance, the entire family immediately responded by saying they wanted all aggressive measures to be continued.

The wife, in the mist of all the talk and noise, sat quietly with her hand on her cheek looking at the floor as if there was something that caught her eye. Her eyes were fatigued with bags that had slowly formed under her eyes over the past couple of days. Her purse hung over her left shoulder but had slid down partly, but she seemed oblivious to the possibility that it may fall. She was older as well, about late seventies I gathered. She had on a long sleeve purple sweater on with off white pants and had those comfortable off white shoes that most folks her age tend to enjoy. Her hair was white and slightly disheveled from sleeping on the long couch next to her husband.

The family continued to talk amongst one another while she sat quietly. Finally, her son finally asked, "what do you think mom?"

Now as a mother and a wife, how would you respond? Here you have your husband who is sick as he can be and looking miserable and on the other hand you have most of the family saying that aggressive measures should be continued. Going against the majority vote can have long term effects and may break some family ties, while going with the vote may prolong your husband's misery. I felt terrible for her. I felt terrible for her husband who could not say a single word and be part of this terrible time. At this very moment, I felt like yelling and saying "have you all seen a code blue? Not on television, in real life? Do you have any idea what it feels like to put a tube down or press on an old man's chest? Do you know what it feels like when you feel ribs breaking while you do compressions?"

I had to stay professional and hold in my emotions. All I could do was remember the patient when he came into the hospital. He was a tall African American man who really loved football. On admission, he was having trouble breathing, but he was on less oxygen but still having some trouble. I had managed to make him laugh in the ER. He was a Kansas City Chiefs fan and I am a Chicago Bears fan; so we shared our misery. He was very kind and I shook his hand prior to leaving the room to finalize my orders and he held my hand longer as I started to make my way out and said "thanks doc for taking care of me." Those words, that touch, truly fill your heart with gratitude and remind you why you have chosen to be a physician. At the time it seemed simple, start antibiotics, start some fluids, fix electrolytes, and follow him the next day.

But, soon he became weaker and the infection spread as his immune system was weak and the infection was resistant to many antibiotics. The antibiotics in themselves started to stress and injure his kidneys. Everything started to go backwards. This is why when people ask in the ER, "how long is my husband going to be in the hospital?" The answer to this is always uncertain. I think we tend to ignore the fact that we are human beings and all the advancements in medicine can never one hundred percent predict any hospital course. We are all created in unique ways with the same end result whether it is one year from now or fifty years from now; it is not a matter of if but when.

His wife slowly looked up at my staff with tearing eyes, gave a quick glance towards her family, and then said "I guess we all want to continue aggressive measures. So do what you have to do to keep him alive." She then stood up and asked to be excused from the room.

Later that afternoon, my worst nightmare became true. He stopped breathing. A code blue was called, which triggered several nurses and doctors to flood the room. I ran in and began telling anesthesia and everyone about the patient so we all get informed of why he most likely stopped breathing. We started the code and I started chest compressions as he had no pulse. With each chest compression my eyes were flooded with tears. I could not hold them back. Thank God for my glasses and the mask we had to wear because the patient was in isolation given the type of infection he had. I felt his ribs crack with each chest compression; his head bopping with each forceful compression. His eyes were rolled over to the side, his limbs flailing in synch with my compressions, and his lips started to turn blue as we bagged him and ultimately placed a metal tube down his throat with a bag over it to continue oxygenation. After several minutes, we were ready to rush him to the medical ICU. I slipped my mask off my mouth and watched the bed roll down the hallway with people running behind holding bags of fluid and IV lines. I threw my gloves in the trash can and began the lonely walk down the hallway towards the family waiting room.

While I walked, I was filled with several emotions involving sadness, anger, and full of questions if there was anything I could have done to prevent this result. I arrived at the waiting room to meet his wife, who by this time was aware of what had happened given all the noise and people that had flooded his room. I briefed them as to what had happened and that he was moved to the medical ICU. They appreciated this conversation and made their way to the ICU. As the doors of the waiting room closed behind them, I plopped down on a chair and stared at the empty wall. I began to think what I would want to be done if I had metastatic cancer and my wife was sitting at bedside. I was saddened by the thought of my wife having to be in that situation and watch me suffer. It is at this very moment I appreciated the value of advanced directives and the importance of talking about dying early with our loved ones. As much as we may not enjoy the conversation, it is a reality we must face and discuss with all of our family members very clearly. The stress of the hospital can place quite a burden on our resident physicians. It is these experiences, questions, and emotions that challenge every resident. At times, the resident may not realize the emotional burden upon them until they go home or their personal stress threshold is overwhelmed to a breaking point. It is important to recognize situations when emotions start to build, because management and organization of these emotions will prevent emotional collapse. Unfortunately, it is not only the stress of the hospital that haunts and challenges each and every resident; it is the financial burden that follows our resident physicians for years to come.

CHAPTER 9

Ridiculous Financial Burden

It is absolutely amazing how expensive graduate education is becoming. Where is the incentive to seek graduate education? In an economy where a college education may not open up enough doors and the applicant is told to seek graduate studies, one must weigh the risks and benefit of such a pursuit. In my training I was surprised by the number of people who had no idea what it took to become a medical resident. Furthermore, some did not know what a medical resident entailed. So, very briefly, after 4 years of college, each applicant must take the MCAT, which is a standardized test used to weed out applicants during medical school admissions process. Once the exam is completed, an application to medical school must be submitted. It is important to understand that this application process is very expensive. The application itself may have fifty to two hundred dollars in fees. Given the competition of medical school admission, each applicant on average applies to about five to ten medical schools if not more. So now we are in the thousands of dollars in expenses. Then the medical school invites the candidate for an interview which requires travel expenses such as hotel, food, transport, to attend these interviews.

Once you are accepted from a medical school, most medical students take on student loans to afford this education. Most medical students will enter medical school with college loans already and are accruing interest on these loans. It is impossible to expect medical students to be working while getting medical education given the competitive nature of the education. So their loans not only include just tuition, books, and laptop or other equipment, but also living expense. Medical students take the USMLE or COMLEX which are standardized medical exams for allopathic and osteopathic medical license respectively. These exams have three steps and each step costs close to six hundred dollars. Most medical students will take a review course from Kaplan or other companies which will cost them another few hundred dollars. By their third year in medical school, one applies to residency programs. This will cost them another few thousand of dollars. Again, they are invited for interviews which come with a cost. The average loan for incoming medical resident is close to $250,000.

Most medical residents are married as well and may have children. The average income for a medical resident is about $43,000. It becomes evident that it is impossible to make any loan payments during residency; thus, these loans go into forbearance, which means you do not have to make payments but interest continues to accrue on the principle balance. I must admit, watching this principal balance rise steadily over the years makes your heart race and fear ultimately overcomes confidence. This fear can not only consume the resident but can also have a profound effect on marriage and the entire social system that supports each single resident.

I was married to my wife in June 2007. We had moved to Kansas City within days after our marriage to start a new life, new job, and a new place for both of us. It was a steep mountain whose terrain was not familiar to us. This mountain had a few rest stops along the way and we met people who would give us advice, but it had little effect on us as we were unsure how to apply it to this journey we had never taken before. We had packed our belongings, said our goodbyes to family and friends, and started up this mountain. The climate surrounding this mountain was also variable. We had to adjust to the cold winters and winds that would almost blow us off track or even off the mountain. There were times I would consider getting off this grueling mountain, but the financial burden was too great. How could I pay close to $300,000 back in a reasonable amount of time with any other job? This would be a terrible decision for me, and more importantly, my family. I had to do this for them. So I continued.

We had to live small. Each grocery list was reviewed thoroughly and asked ourselves, "do we really need this right now?" It took time to organize the expenses and devise a strategic plan to prepare for this catastrophic payback that awaited us upon graduation. This is a difficult task. It requires planning for three years down the road. More importantly, it truly affects your professional satisfaction because this debt weighs on your shoulders for the next several years. What is worse is if you do not have a plan, then it can bury you. Unfortunately, this also deeply wounds resident morale and also future medical school applicants. People are weighing the cost and benefit of pursuing a medical education. Moreover, people who do graduate from medical school are seeking specialist positions to make more money; leaving primary care in the dust. As reimbursement continues to decline for physicians, residents are less likely to seek primary care, which is clearly evident in our enormous primary care shortage. Furthermore, the primary care physicians are being forced to see more patients in less amount of time, which only compromises patient care. The incentives are not in the right place. The profession is being attacked from every direction and residents become consumed by it because they are not prepared for it. This leads to a number of physicians who are in terrible financial situations because they simply did not plan ahead financially. Furthermore, they did not know how to manage their salaries once they graduated.

I was blessed to find a financial planner who helped us organize our debts, formulate a plan, and implement a daily routine to prepare for the future. My wife was the administrator for the house and took care of our monthly budget. There is so much paperwork with student loans, applications, and bills that we had to set up folders, bins, to organize and assure not to miss deadlines. In reflecting upon this difficult time, I am saddened by how much stress residency placed on my wife. Furthermore, little do people realize that they are the ones that also sacrifice alongside the resident. The lonely nights, the few phone calls during the day, the lonely dinners, the lack of any meaningful vacation or travel for three solid years is just a start. Hearing stories about her friends' travels and vacations always saddened me. I kept telling myself, when all this is done, I will take her on the best vacations possible, but in the meantime, I had to be patient. She would be on the phone laughing and enjoying their stories only to replay the entire story to me over dinner in a theatrical way. I would listen and enjoy her laughter; her colorful way of describing and sharing stories is always entertaining.

At times, I was so tired that just keeping my eyes open was difficult. My feet would be swollen. My heart would be full of emotion relating to the multiple patient and family interactions from the day and my mind racing with thoughts ranging from science to concerns about us. These were the ingredients for the nightly collapse on my couch only to be awakened at midnight by my wife to come to bed. I would stumble over and collapse on the bed again with my wife's' voice in the background whispering, "I love you."

The financial burden of a medical education must be addressed in all medical schools and residency programs. Financial planners need to mobilize and help these students. Programs across the country need to take this burden under consideration as it impacts not only the individual student, but the medical profession. Young physicians today are more in debt than their predecessors. More pressure is being placed on efficiency and the dynamics of the health care industry is changing so fast that these young physicians have no clue how to keep up. More importantly, when they graduate and enter higher tax brackets, they have no idea how to manage their salaries; ultimately swallowing them up in an enormous financial crisis. This may lead to divorce, misguided children, or even patient care as each patient encounter becomes tainted with concerns of reimbursement.

We need to go back to the basics and learn from our past. Being a physician is a privilege and an honor to have the ability to take care of people in their most vulnerable state. We have a huge responsibility with each individual and all of humanity. The system must support and nurture this culture and bring back the environment where decisions are not disturbed by reimbursement rates, student loans, or the politics of Washington. Capitalism is attempting to swallow our health care system and it simply will destroy it if it prevails. Let's be honest, we have all seen and witnessed greedy physicians who boast about their earnings or do unnecessary procedures to support their Ferraris or Jaguars. Have we all lost our focus here? Who is to blame?

CHAPTER 10

Where Are The Incentives?

I have been privileged to witness the evolution of medicine. I watched my mom practice medicine in the late 1980's evolve into the present state of medicine. It has gone from the paternal patient-physician relationship to a more dynamic individualistic relationship where both parties share knowledge to establish a treatment plan. The paternal-physician dynamic is referred to a relationship where patients trusted their physicians and looked at their physician as the ultimate authority in treating them. The partnership dynamic, which is more present today, is where the patient and physician work together to arrive at the diagnosis. The advent of the internet and other resources has empowered patients to research their condition prior to their clinic visit. This can make the clinic visit become longer. However, in a time where efficiency and number of patients seen are the foundation for the financial stability of any outpatient clinic, where are the incentives to allow time for a discussion to occur? The current system does not provide incentives for patients and physicians to simply sit and discuss their illness without a timer hovering above their head.

Reimbursement rates have declined, health care is being bought by corporate organizations, there is cessation of solo practice simply because no one can afford it, the rise of 'minute clinics' which is competing with primary care groups across the country, the value of primary care has diminished, physicians are working more hours and seeing more patients in less amount of time, and finally hospitals are becoming larger with more beds increasing the demands of its physicians. Meanwhile, as a society, we are aging, have more co-morbidity and living unhealthy lifestyles; largely because the incentives in this country focus on working and making money more than spending time with family and on self-improvement. In this evolving climate we demand more from our physicians. For example, we expect our physicians to be knowledgeable of current research, provide more time, be available at minutes' notice, and provide the single most efficient care possible.

If we pause and reflect on this dynamic climate of health care, it becomes evident the enormous amount of stress today's physician is in and how unprepared our young physicians are to approach this climate. Should we not invest more in our health care starting with our young physicians? Should we not invest more in them because after all, they will be the ones that will take care of humanity? They are the ones who may possibly allow us to live longer with a quality of life that we perceive to be appropriate for ourselves? Instead of spending millions of dollars in entertainment, which is clearly getting out of hand in this country, critical entities that significantly impact our daily lives are completely being ignored. Make no mistake, I love watching NFL, NBA, movies, and Colbert Report. But, I find it unbearable to tolerate the number of uninsured people in America and the quality of care a super power is providing for its own people in some of these communities. The time to make a change is now for the betterment of the American people.

We all have seen the charts where the United States is depicted as one of the most obese nations in the world (see http://www.cdc.gov/obesity/data/adult.html). In comparison to rest of the countries, we rank extremely low in survival and high in infant mortality (see cdc.gov). How could that be with all the technological advances we have made? As a society, we have to go back to the basics. Exercise and diet must be rewarded in some fashion – tax breaks, discounts on gym memberships with employment, allow time to go to the gym, healthier cafeteria food in schools, and reduction of the cost of living. The American culture has allowed work to dominate our existence. This is clearly demonstrated by the fact that people are retiring at a later age because they simply cannot afford to retire any sooner. How is this not worrisome? How have we allowed the cost of living to become so expensive?

Just writing this makes me smile, because there is no way we would ever agree to this! Imagine McDonalds saying, "ok we will stop selling our burgers for the betterment of the American people." The mighty dollar always prevails. Is this how it's supposed to be? We turn the other way when we know there an obesity epidemic in this country and allow corporations to make billions off of the very foods that are killing us as a society? It simply does not make sense.

So where are the incentives for us as a society to live a healthier lifestyle? When will people understand that we literally are killing ourselves? We have allowed ourselves to justify reasons for not watching our diet and implementing an exercise regimen into our daily activities. Work dominates our daily routine such that fitting in a workout seems like an impossible mission. Changing the

American culture now is difficult. We have already lost the battle of preserving family and personal time. Work has already consumed that aspect of our lives. Thus, it is our personal responsibility to adjust our daily activities around an exercise program. An hour of activity a day is all that it takes. More importantly, it is critical that we change our diet. Since when did quantity become more important that quality in the American restaurant industry? The American people have allowed this to happen. It is our own fault for allowing the portions to become larger; thus, we are over-eating on a daily basis. If the American people fought this transformation by not buying these foods or going to these restaurants, it would have changed behavior. But we didn't. The "All You Can Eat" buffets continue to be busy and "super size" still remains an option.

If we allowed this culture to grow, then how can one not expect a rise in chronic illnesses? It becomes obvious that if such a culture is supported then there must be growth and support for health care providers to take care of our growing obesity epidemic. The health care system has to provide incentives for preventative services. There should have been an urgent and aggressive calling for primary care physicians. Federal and state programs should have been created to provide incentives for primary care offices to spend time with these patients in attempts to keep them away from the ER. A clinic visit is much cheaper than a hospital visit. All this would have made sense. But we didn't do it. We stood silent and watched as people filled their stomachs with large portions of greasy meals. Our children grew larger only to die before their mothers eyes. The cost to keep our society alive is obviously more expensive given the obesity epidemic. Did we expect anything different?

CHAPTER 11

Rising Cost of Health Care
Is No Surprise!

As health care evolves, we have seen many changes take place. We are quick to marvel at the new toys that fill our radiology suites and our cath labs; drool over the robots that are now assisting in surgery. But, do we ever stop and think about what has happened to that basic fundamental role of physicians, nurses, techs, and other health care providers? We have obviously found novel ways to gather more information, but what about managing that information? Surely, as information becomes more complex, the comprehension and management of that information must also become more difficult. So, how has this affected our health care providers and how have they responded?

When a patient comes to the ER with shortness of breath or even chest pain, there are a host of orders that go into action. Evidence based practice has improved outcomes and definitely has improved survival, but it has also significantly increased the amount of protocols each hospital now practices. These protocols are order sets on a sheet of paper filled with boxes and spaces where physicians can fill in the blanks for any orders that they wish to order that goes beyond the order set. These order sets in a sense provide an algorithm if you will, which he/she will select to assure the standard of care is delivered.

For example, if a patient has chest pain, then the order set would include an aspirin, certain medications, an electrocardiogram, a host of blood draws, a chest xray, and a cardiology consult. So, even though a patients clinical symptoms may be inconsistent with a myocardial infarction (heart attack), then the order set simply is a waste of money. However, not initiating the protocol can raise several questions if the patient did have a atypical presentation and ended up having a heart attack, or the agencies that measure quality will raise several concerns as to why the protocol was not initiated; eliminating the opportunity for the hospital to win any type of local/national recognition. Thus, the incentives are not in the right place to reducing the cost of health care.

It becomes evident that physicians must be aware of these protocols, initiate them when appropriate, and must be prepared to justify why or why not they used the protocols. This is where all the bureaucrats get all excited and several meetings will take place; frustrating and taking away the pure enjoyment of the practice of medicine.

When a physician takes care of a single patient, there are a number of complex interactions and processes that take place all at once. Let's just take a moment to look at all the forces at play in this interaction. First off, we have the physician stepping into the room and interviewing the patient and begin his/her investigative work. As the two individuals converse, certain questions are asked and responses are analyzed, while the physicians eyes scan the patients movements, gestures, and their speech; all at the same time. Family members are usually the audience in the background; intermittently sneaking in a comment or two during this conversation. At times, family members are able to relate the "actual" events when a patient tries to minimize the significance of their symptoms. Finally, when the physician decides on the treatment plan, he/she sits to write orders. The patient has the expectation that whatever they just revealed to the physician, they will analyze the data and find some solution to their illness.

When the physician sits to write orders, now he/she enters the expectations of the organization where they must fill out the right forms to meet standard of care. National guidelines and professional expectations are intertwined with the organizations in this step. Meanwhile, it is imperative to keep cost in mind as well. But, failure to follow certain protocols or the practice of defensive medicine can raise costs significantly.

After completing the orders, the treatment plan for the patient begins. The following days, the physician must coordinate care with nurses, techs, and consultants to provide the best care. All the while, there are care coordinators who count the hospital days. It is all too familiar to any physician when they get a page from these individuals and the discussion starts with, "I was looking through Mr. Joe's chart and…" This is followed by the physicians explanation as to why the patient has to stay in the hospital for the next couple of days. Sometimes this is not a problem, but there are times where this is frustrating.

Therefore, the role of physicians is moving beyond simply patient care. As quality and accreditation agencies work together in assuring the best health care is being implemented in our hospitals, physicians are recognized as the integral employees of hospitals who can illustrate to these agencies the hospitals mission to provide the best health care possible. Thus, the physician becomes the symbol, the deliverer, and the illustration of the mission of any health care organization. So, it follows then, that health care organizations across America must recognize the importance of their physicians and work towards closing the communication gap between administration and physicians. The best health care organizations are those where physicians are actively involved in administration. There is a symbiotic relationship that exists between administration and its medical staff. Each entity exists and succeeds as long as the other does the same. Moreover, the patient and their families, have become increasingly a significant component of a health care organizations' success and mere existence.

Patient satisfaction surveys, the internet, and simply the word of mouth dictate what kind of reputation a health care organization achieves. Therefore, patients, in a sense, have incredible power in affecting the business of any health care organization or provider. The internet provides an endless audience for one to either compliment or criticize any health care provider or organization. This power and responsibility is critical for the American people to understand and appreciate. With power comes greater responsibility. Thus, before we hit send on any blog or website, we must stop and think about what we are about to say about our health care providers or organizations before the message enters the cyber world. Physicians, administrators, and patients should work together to make the delivery of health care most efficient and effective.

I noted this intricate web of relationships in the delivery of health care early in my career. To my dismay, I must admit I have found patients who abuse their role and responsibility to a point where much discussion and deliberation must take place in attempts to maintain efficient delivery. The sad part is that these interactions take so much administrative time, that it takes time away and may compromise the health care delivery of other patients in the hospital. It is too common in academic hospitals where we have the "usual suspects" who come to the ER with vague complaints and seek pain medications. As residents, we do what we are told and so we admit these patients only to have multiple arguments and discussions regarding IV pain medications the following morning. Today, pain has received such national attention that it is becoming more difficult to accurately assess drug seeking behavior versus true pain.

As residents, we all remember those patients who can truly put on a show with tears, the wails of cries, and then the aggressive behavior that prompts a call for security. In these interactions, the physician becomes a detective; observing each action and expression, questioning each pain complaint the patient reports. This is unfortunate, but necessary. It is at the time of discharge where the common question from an abuser that leaves all physicians a sick feeling in their stomach: "I ran out of all my medications, including my pain medications, can you write me a script for all the meds?" The real loser in all of this is the one who truly has pain and finds themselves proving they have reason to be in pain.

So, I believe the role of physicians is to be team leaders. They must lead a team of multidisciplinary specialists to provide the most efficient care possible. To illustrate this, the physician must guide the social worker and case manager towards what needs the patient has, educate the family and the patient regarding the illness they have, work with nursing staff to assure orders are executed with efficiency and accuracy, and finally, working with administration in reducing hospital days and providing excellent health care by following all measures of standard of care; thus, adding value to the health care organization. We must make this transition from individual to team approach. Unfortunately, I still see moments where physicians do not converse with physicians and the chart becomes the only means of communication. Moreover, I still see miscommunication between physicians and nurses. How is this possible? Well, one clear reason is that hospitals are busier than ever and patient load and acuity is significantly higher. This demands determination and dedication by all health care providers to make special effort in building bridges for communication to take place effectively.

Team rounds are a simple solution. If the nurse, physician, pharmacist, social worker, and case manager all round together would be great. However, emergencies happen, some family have more questions than others, and there are various other factors that can slow this process and make it inefficient. Thus, it is critical for the organization to be creative in formulating creative solutions, buy-in and determination from physicians, and cooperation from patient and family members to facilitate efficient morning rounds. An efficient electronic record can make rounds even more efficient. Real time data at the bedside can significantly facilitate efficient decision making at the bedside. So, instead of investing in nice furniture in the waiting room or big signs boosting about ones achievements, hospitals across America should invest in the most efficient electronic record.

As I practice Internal Medicine as a staff physician, I have experienced working in hospitals that have a great EMR and those that still live in the "old days" with paper charts and minimal electronic record. I would argue that quality and delivery of effective health care is far greater in an institution with an efficient and thorough electronic record. Besides, most young physicians are being trained in setting where sophisticated electronic records are utilized.

Thus, it is less likely that they will seek employment in hospitals that have anything less than what they were trained using. It is critical that administrators realize this and also the old physicians who are resistant to change; bottom line is, if we want more efficient health care and want to recruit and retain the brightest minds to work at our hospitals, then we must provide the resources that will facilitate their practice.

Thus, a clear role for physicians is to promote the establishment of an efficient electronic record. Physicians must play an active role in the production and implementation of such a system. It must be user friendly and able to withstand future modifications and upgrades. I still hear disgruntled staff mumble their disgust for the electronic record. The young physicians are seen as a threat to their way of practice. It is all too common for a young physician to hear comments like, "you have it easy. Back in the old days, we had to rely on our hands, eyes, and ears to make a diagnosis." Although this may be true, the complexity of health care today is far greater than the "old days." The number of co morbidities, the rise in unhealthy lifestyle, and the lack of insurance pose a different climate for today's physician to practice. I would argue, both populations have their own challenges as times change; no population faced a greater challenge than the other. Each physician today trained in a different era and thus possesses skills that the other may lack. Thus, it becomes imperative that these two generations of physicians work together to deliver the most effective and efficient health care.

CHAPTER 12

Life Outside The Hospital

One of the most challenging aspects of any profession is balancing work and life. We spend countless number of years preparing for the achievement of a certain profession; making several sacrifices, reminding ourselves that the achievement of a certain profession will make those sacrifices worthwhile. To make matters more complicated, usually we are accompanied by our loved ones who will tag along and follow our passion in hopes that once the goal is met, life will automatically unfold the way we had hoped. All the struggles that we face along this journey are painted with the hope that the end result will eliminate the fatigue we endured along the way. However, once we stand there holding our degree in one hand and look out towards our loved ones, what do we find? More importantly, when we are in our most quiet and private moment in our life, what do our reflections entail?

For me, I find that much time has been lost. A medical degree is a brutal struggle that once it is achieved, one finds themselves tired and thirsty for a "normal life." We want to be able to go to family gatherings, spend vacation time, come home earlier than 5pm on a daily basis, and have weekends free to spend with family. However, this is not true.

Upon graduation from residency, the responsibilities increase exponentially. Student loans consume our budget. This initiates the need to work extra hours, work the extra weekends, and focus on production every quarter of the year. If one plans to buy a home or any other asset, it must be balanced with the debt that hangs overhead. It takes financial discipline to mobilize financial resources towards reducing this debt, instead of spending on vacation and other pleasures. Graduation and the start of a staff position almost makes one feel that they need to splurge a bit, but one must stay patient and assess their financial fitness. This is where the trouble lies. Once young physicians see their paychecks and the bank account increase tremendously, it requires efficient wealth management to prevent worsening debt. The real question is whether we are preparing our young physicians to manage their wealth efficiently?

I have seen many families and individuals who poorly managed their wealth. They feel this expectation and demand from others to suddenly become a successful wealthy physician. So the disastrous behavior begins with the purchase of unnecessarily big houses, cars, etc; raising their debt significantly like a tsunami that gently rises before it splashes over a town within seconds. As young physicians make their purchases and manage their debt, their loved ones are also in this struggle with them. I think every loving husband/wife desires to somehow reward their spouse who has sacrificed and struggled with them through the brutal years of training. However, responsibilities remain and one must balance this with recreational spending.

It takes team work to efficiently and effectively balance work and life. It is a partnership between loved ones to assure their vision is met. A vision is set in every household, whether we sit and draw it out or established through discussions and mutually understood over time. For my wife and I our vision is to live with minimal debt or debt free if possible. Family is the central focus at all times. Any decisions that are made must consider that essential question, how will my decision affect my family? This means, funds must be set aside for children, their education, basic house and livable expenses, and balance recreational expenses – never splurging so much that it strains our budget. There are ways to set aside money so that recreational shopping can be done and not affect the overall budget. Creative solutions will keep the vision in site for any household. Financial fitness is a huge player in balancing work and life; if the finances are maintained and strong, then feelings of frustration, anger, and resentment are kept at a minimum and professional satisfaction is at a maximum.

Young physicians have other motivations other than their financial needs to work hard and maybe put in a few extra hours. Once you are a staff physician, it is an incredible feeling of achievement, but also responsibility. The days of calling another physician to verify your decisions are gone and you are pushed forward as a leader of the treatment team. Now it is your responsibility to efficiently manage the health of a patient. Every decision you make is assessed against multiple standards, and protocols. Discussions regarding your decisions will begin the minute you make them. This is a tremendous amount of responsibility. If one is not ready for this role, they find themselves questioning themselves multiple times, maybe rounding on patients multiple times in a day. This may threaten their perceived competency from their colleagues or other health professionals; ultimately, placing more stress onto their loved ones as days at work will undoubtedly get longer. Moreover, an unprepared young physician will likely take their frustrations out at home than at work, compromising their support system even more.

On the other hand, those who are prepared for the responsibility and enjoy the leadership roles they have finally achieved find themselves satisfied with their work. Moreover, when loved ones see the satisfaction, it reduces their stress and brings a sense of achievement. As one grows in their profession, undoubtedly physicians are in a position where they can make significant changes in another human beings life. In treating a patient, or even managing a complex case efficiently, leaving the patient and family satisfied with your work, this opens the gate for compliments. It is not uncommon for any physician to be thanked for their work, which is much appreciated. However, for some, it only hardens their soul and swells their head – you can almost see their heads swell in front of you as you compliment them. Then there are those who stay humble and divert the compliments to the entire treatment team as we have already established, the practice of medicine is a team sport.

Praise provides any human being a sense of good feeling and motivates them to work towards obtaining more praise. Similarly, when one gambles, the reward is cherished and the search for more begins. In the same way, the practice of medicine can be addicting. When one makes the right decision in critical moments or treats a patient where the patient recovers, feelings of satisfaction can lead to addiction; facilitating longer work hours and time away from family. This is a toxin that must be recognized by every physician and managed before it consumes them. Researchers are dedicated to their work, but what about their families? Is it good that we praise world renown researchers who work 24/7 and place their names and pictures on posters illustrating dedication? Is this dedication managed properly?

I would argue, the one who manages their time and balances their work with family is the real dedicated worker. Some of us work to gain praise, fame, or some monetary reward. Thus, one finds themselves working to satisfy these pleasures. However, in my experience, these people are never satisfied because the thirst for more is far greater and powerful than anything that is sought to quench it. The reality is, corporations, hospitals, and other health care establishments will motivate and encourage any physician that brings them more business. So, all the smiles and gifts that you may get from administration must be taken with caution. Greed is an evil that preys on those who seek reward and gratification for their work, instead of professional development. We must, as physicians, keep our morality in check. Although we do participate in a capitalistic society where capital gains are put on a pedestal, the business of medicine has a human component that cannot be forgotten.

Businesses can replace their employees anytime and will if production is not meeting their goals. In the same way, hospitals are no different in following suit. Thus, it is important to realize that familial love is genuine, pure, and unconditional. The question remains, how do we train our future physicians to take on these challenges of the ever changing health care in not only the United States, but the rest of the world?

CHAPTER 13

Advice for Medical School Educators

The main problem in today's medical education is that we have lost focus. We need to go back to the basics. Technology, the speed of medical advancements, and the complexity of patient care has completely thrown us off track. There has been the introduction of powerpoint slides filled with text which the lecturer simply reads, then the laptops, to no more textbooks! I remember when I was on rounds one day and our staff had asked one of the students if they own a textbook on physical exam – the infamous Mosby's. His reply was simply, "Oh yeah, it's online." That didn't go well with our staff who had more than forty years of experience and was the father of physical exam at our hospital. Books have lost their worth these days. So, this section is to re-focus us back to the basics and hopefully can add some value back into medical training.

We must admit that our medical schools do a pretty good job in training our students the basic sciences of anatomy, physiology, biochemistry, and pharmacology. Several physicians teach these classes and share some personal experiences during these lectures that add value to the subject at hand. Medical schools across the country are adding more facilities to boast about their anatomy labs, interactive and technologically advanced classrooms, and certainly the statistics on board pass rates are screamed through a megaphone whenever possible. Financial assistance offices stand ready to offer multiple solutions for them to obtain their ridiculous tuition fees and are willing to provide banks with the opportunity to provide student loans to cover those large tuitions; negating the burden they are about to place on their own students. How cost-effective are our medical schools? We must stand back and ask the question, are medical schools deserving of all this cash reward and glory they claim?

One may argue that medical schools simply reinforce the sciences that have already been introduced to the student, thus making positive results inevitable. Medical knowledge is simply added to a foundation that has already been placed from pre-med courses prior to entering medical school. So, it follows then, the glory that some medical schools receive, is it because of the quality of education they provide or is it the fact that they attract some of the brightest students who have a solid base from prestigious colleges?

Some of the brightest students we have usually have taken a course in anatomy or physiology prior to their first year of medical school. So, it is not the case that they are exposed to completely brand new literature and information; there is some familiarity to the content. Most premedical students major in biology or chemistry even today, which further limits their overall knowledge base. Many medical schools promote or motivate applicants to major in subjects other than science; however, by in large most continue to major in the sciences. So, what can students do to broaden their knowledge base? What should program directors do at medical schools? And finally, how do we continue that process in residency when time seems to be in competition with multiple responsibilities?

These are tough questions to answer and must invite a thorough discussion. If we start with the admission process, we can begin to discuss the types of students medical schools attract. There are some rumors out there that medical schools are becoming more interested in applicants that major in subjects other than the sciences. I think this is a good thing. Once students enter medical school, they are taught nothing but science. So college is the time when students have the ability to learn about world socioeconomics, history, culture, political science, communication studies, finance, mathematics, etc. We need to cultivate well rounded students to enter the field of medicine. The world is becoming more diverse with various ideologies. How can we prepare health care leaders if they cannot understand or influence the rest of the world, let alone their own communities?

Once these students are accepted, our coursework in medical schools can certainly improve. Today, we teach physiology, anatomy, biochemistry, and the rest of the sciences in the first two years of medical school. Sure, there are the physical exam classes and ethics classes that are thrown in the mix towards the end of their years. But I see the problem in two major ways. One, we must teach students the importance of understanding the physiology of the human body in such a way that the complexity is appreciated. It is quite fascinating how the human body is interconnected. Most of us take each organ, even each cell in our body for granted. The medical student of all people must gain the appreciation and respect for the human body. In a culture where each discovery becomes a business opportunity, one must not lose their fundamental principles as a physician; that is to focus on improving the health of their patients, their communities, and ultimately the world.

Empathy must we instilled in our students such that they will never lose that ability to feel their patients pain and suffering. As a society, we must allow these students and physicians to continue to be empathic. What happens is those negative interactions with patients or family members, can certainly cloud ones ability to empathize and unfortunately may lead to the inability to empathize. We cannot let this happen to our physicians. So it becomes our job as teachers and mentors to assure our students maintain that ability to empathize and look past any negative attitudes or forces that may threaten this vital component of our profession.

In addition, our students are surrounded by such tremendous debt, how do we maintain their focus on the patient without thinking about repayment? This is the challenge of our present day medical student. How do we allow them to enjoy primary care in a world where specialists are more financially rewarded? This is the issue. If we can get our medical students to appreciate and respect the true essence of the human body and what it means to be a physician, while blocking all the negative attitudes that come with poor reimbursement, long hours, student debt, and the constant stress that comes with patient care. How do we do that? Again, that is the challenge of medical schools to find staff that stimulate the minds of their students and prepare them to cope with these negative forces. Sure, medicine is a business and one must be able to participate to survive. But, this does not justify any physician from losing their empathy and their fundamental core in the practice of medicine. We have been too lenient with this crucial element with policy-makers. We must re-focus and protect the practice from being consumed by greedy capitalistic monsters that salivate over the opportunities that exist in the practice of health care. How can we allow pharmaceutical companies to charge so much for medications? How can we allow our own people the inability to afford medications that will improve survival? It is no surprise we rank towards the bottom in the terms of survival when compared with the rest of the world; despite spending the most in the world on health care!

The second part of this problem is how do we communicate this complexity to the general public? This can be done in group discussions as well as by the lecturer. There needs to be more group work in medical school, where students are required to lead discussions and work together to find solutions. In the real world, this is what is done on a daily basis. As a staff physician, I lead several teams in a single day. It is critical to be able to get people together, like the case manager, social worker, and others to gain insight as to the best discharge plan for the patient. Similarly, in dealing with a complex case involving multiple specialists, one must be able to facilitate a discussion with all specialists together to come up with the best solution. Believe me, when one is managing several specialists it is not only managing the medical issues at hand, but also various egos and personalities; which can be difficult at times.

The second major problem in our medical school training is that not enough time is spent on the business of medicine. How to start a practice? How does billing work? What is proper coding? When we teach our medical students how to write progress notes, why not teach them about level of care and proper documentation to fulfill that level of care? This way, students learn how to properly document for coding purposes, but also how to communicate their thought processes to other members of the treatment team by writing a thorough note.

Health finance must enter our medical school curriculum. An introduction to the topics will at least familiarize students with the language so that when they take on leadership positions in the hospitals, they can understand financial documents and are better prepared for making informed decisions. Management, human resources, and marketing all must become part of the curriculum. Majority of the hospitals are moving towards a team approach. Moreover, we must encourage students for office based practices and primary care. We are in desperate need of primary care physicians in this country. One way to encourage students towards primary care is teaching them the team work, coordination, and leadership that are involved in primary care. Moreover, when physicians start an office practice, they are business owners of that practice. So, we must introduce, encourage, and show the great benefits of being a business owner. If students become more comfortable with business language and ideas, the more they will move towards participating in one.

Understanding how policy is made will allow medical students and future physicians to efficiently influence the policy making process. Policy is what makes health care reform. It is the foundation of how change is even possible. So how can we expect our young physicians to influence policy change if they don't understand where to start? Thus, part of the second year curriculum must include some lectures and exercises on public policy. Again, group discussions where students and share their knowledge of an existing problem, but coming together for potential solutions is an effective way to teach policy. We also need more collaboration between health departments and medical schools. Students must gain an understanding of who are the players in our health department. Physicians and the health department must work together to change communities. Thus, it makes sense to form bridges early in medical training. In addition, this experience may stimulate some students towards primary care. There are a tremendous amount of leadership opportunities for future physicians. We simply have to make them comfortable to be leaders and equip them with fundamental language so they can actively participate.

How many of us met physicians who are incredibly smart, but cannot communicate? Or, how many of us met medical students who are brilliant, but shy away from leadership opportunities because they get nervous in front of people? Why are we not investing in providing these brilliant students with resources and skills that would encourage them to take on leadership projects? This is the problem with today's health care. The fundamental development of a future physician is the training we get in medical school. If we do not teach these basic skills and educate them about management, marketing, finance, and communication studies, how can we expect any change?

These courses should be taught in year two of medical school. These courses should be spread out instead of being taught at the trail end of their second year of medical school. Even in the first year of medical school, some of this training can start. The idea is to get the student mentally prepared to be a physician. They must be educated from the beginning that the goal of medical school is not just passing exams or board exams; the goal is to be the best physician they can be. This is their business and they are in control of the end product. The medical school should do whatever it can to provide the resources via community partnerships with the health department and long term care facilities, interactive classes, and providing an environment where leadership is encouraged and minds are constantly challenged outside of the basic sciences. The student then has the ultimate responsibility to soak up all this knowledge and personalize their approach to the practice of medicine.

CHAPTER 14

Advice for the

Medical Student

One of the greatest investments and decisions I made during my medical training was getting my Masters in Health Administration. At the time, the weekend classes and the night classes were tough, but upon completion, it has significantly enriched my career. Knowledge equips you with confidence and allows you to maximize your strengths. It will open doors that once may have been closed. More importantly, it facilitates a better understanding of the health care you provide to your patients. It is ultimately the responsibility of the student to seek knowledge, humble themselves in recognizing their weaknesses, and strengthening those weaknesses. When one makes the decision to become a physician, there is more than science to learn: business, politics, and communication are critical topics that need to be learned.

Truth is, medicine is a big business. The first step is to recognize this fact. Early recognition will allow the student to start taking courses in subjects other than biology or chemistry. I would argue that it is the responsibility of colleges to promote this by including some business classes in their pre-med curriculum. I remember taking accounting and finance in college as part of my health administration major and it felt like I was exploring a side of my brain I never thought existed. Accounting and finance were tough classes that required analysis and a thought process similar to medicine, but with some variance.

The analytical approach to real world financial decisions was challenging, yet rewarding when the solution was obtained. The basics of budgeting, costs, revenues, management, human resources, health law, public policy, and communication studies are critical to present day physicians. Certainly, all these topics cannot be taught to every pre-med student as a curriculum in addition to their basic sciences, but at least exposing them to basic finance and accounting as a start should be considered. Public policy is extremely important for any future physicians as it will become part of their career the minute they step into medical school. How policy is formed, evaluating stakeholders, performing a stakeholder analysis, and understanding current issues with an understanding of policy formation are important.

Furthermore, it is important to understand that by simply providing courses does not mean the student will know everything about a subject. For example, by providing courses in finance or accounting does not make a student become a professional financial analyst or an accountant. It simply familiarizes the student with the language so that they can build on this knowledge as they progress in their medical training. In the same way, medical school introduces the student to the language of medicine and disease processes for the student to build on as they progress in their training. So, it is critical that we reassess what we are teaching our pre-med students and ask the question, are we truly preparing these young adults for future medical practice?

Once the student enters medical school, the first year is nerve wrecking and intense. All of a sudden, you are surrounded by other geeks who are just as smar or even smarter than you! The competition becomes quite intense. Conversations become somewhat superficial and it is always hilarious how people will ask around how they did after an exam to reassure themselves that they had marked the right answer. Why do we do this? It's not like we can go back and change the answer! Anyway, we all have things we look back on and laugh at or just shake our head. Life certainly facilitates entertainment. I think that in the first year, the medical student should be exposed to health law, public policy, health finance, and even management. The reason can simply be extrapolated from the previous chapters. Managing a practice, leading a treatment team on the wards, or being an active member of a physician group requires financial and managerial understanding to truly be effective. The biggest handicap our present-day physicians have is the lack of financial and political knowledge such that there cannot be a rational discussion between politicians, administrators, and physicians; simply, because no one understands each other!

The first year, with anatomy, physiology, biochemistry, and the like, it would be to the students' advantage if program directors taught their students basic health administration courses. Once the student advances to the second year, marketing, human resources, and management courses should be taught. After the second year, that student can care less about the classroom because they are off to rotations where they spend all their time in hospitals. Today, health law is taught in the second year just before they go off to their rotation as third year medical students. What is the point of that? We are teaching them one of the most vital courses, whose understanding may ultimately protect them one day, the very last few days of the second year! Who came up with that bright idea! It makes no sense. You must teach students important topics when you have their attention.

At the end of the day, it is the student him/herself who must understand the importance of these subjects. Billions of dollars are pumped into the business of medicine and as a physician you are managing a piece of that business. Each time you enter an exam room, whether it be in a hospital or a clinic, you are marketing yourself, providing a service for revenue, and interacting with ancillary staff that you lead and manage to provide the best health care possible. Now with the advent of social media and various websites to critique physicians, you are evaluated daily. There are reviews about everything, so why not doctors! Therefore, one of the points I made earlier in this book is that our young physicians get inundated with Hollywood stupidity where the physician is suppose to be cool, relaxed, and fun. This has danger written all over it. If you follow suit, it will open a can of worms that you cannot easily control because word today can travel a lot faster and further than ever before. Therefore, one must think a hundred times before they do anything. When you enter the hospital, you are at work, not at home or at some social gathering. You are at work where people depend on you to make the right decisions, to improve their health, and at times, live another day. The cliché "treat patients like your family members" is so true that if taken to heart and implemented, you will automatically conduct honest and effective patient care.

In addition to seeking courses and doing the best you can at educating yourself of various topics, one must take the responsibility towards learning about other health care organizations outside the hospital or the clinic. You see, as students, all we know is what happens in a hospital or a clinic. What about a nursing home, skilled nursing facility, long term acute care facilities, or home health care? Why not allow our students to go over to these facilities and experience what they do on a daily basis. In reality, one must know the qualifications for each facility for insurance to approve care delivered at such facilities. It's too late if we expect our residents to walk over to a skilled nursing facility and learn about them. They rather sleep on their day off!

As alluded to earlier in this book, medical schools can encourage this by having their students do projects or group work that involve these long term care facilities. If these resources are not provided by the medical school, then it becomes the responsibility of the student to seek these opportunities. The bottom line is, that we must not expect schools to provide everything on a silver platter. Again, their main goals as of today are to stay financially viable, continue to grow to encourage more admissions, and of course, have you pass your board exam. Outside of that, why would they care about you? Who cares if you don't understand all the complexities of long term care, understand financial documents, understand how to lead a team of health care providers or communities, or what you decide to do?

This is the problem with our medical schools and our medical students. Each is contributing to the problem in their own way. The schools are focused on the financial gains more than the type of training provided. The students are becoming too dependent on the schools to teach them everything they think they need to know to practice medicine. The practice of medicine is more than board scores, passing exams, even more than your class rank. No one cares for a physician who may be the top of the class and the most brilliant mind in school; but if they cannot utilize those skills towards improving patient care or the health of our communities, what value do they really have?

It is important to recognize that although we teach certain subjects, it is not for certain that the material is understood and implemented 100% each time. Thus, as the student advances to residency, there needs to be an understanding between educators to pass the baton and take over that responsibility.

CHAPTER 15

Advice for the Young Resident

I do not think that there is a single most efficient and effective way to prepare oneself for residency. It is my experience that allows me to reflect and share with my readers some advice that may facilitate a more informed start to residency than I had. In this section I will not only discuss the resident themselves, but also their support system. I think that it is critical that the entire support system, in most cases it entails husband, wife, and loved ones, that must take the time to prepare for the residency years. But first, we must discuss the resident.

The most exciting moment in any medical students' life is the day of graduation. Actually, it is probably the last day of their last rotation, because graduation day is always prolonged and full of boring speeches that are only forgotten the minute we walk away from the venue. It is that special feeling of accomplishment, as if you have just completed the impossible. All the years of studying, memorizing, nerve wrecking exams, restless nights thinking of what specialty you want to pursue, and sacrificing family events to obtain this goal, somehow feels worthwhile.

By the time you are a fourth year medical student, you are accepted at a residency program and are simply counting the days till that first day of residency. You barely pay attention on the last few rotations and find yourself thinking about what you are going to do with your free time while on rounds. Some may even go far as not to care on their last rotations, because the staff at a particular hospital may never see you again anyway; so who cares!

As the days towards residency get closer, the future resident begins to feel nervous. The thoughts of making decisions and being held responsible become nightmares. The reminder of the work hours becomes overwhelming.

It is also during this time that most of your friends who have graduated college may have jobs and possibly in position of growing their families or purchasing their first homes; while you smile with hundreds of thousands of dollars in debt hanging over your head. This can get annoying. You watch people go on trips and make comments of the ridiculous price of medical education; while you justify and remind yourself you did it for a reason.

Most find themselves during these conversations thinking to themselves, "I did make the right decision, right?" At times, some may find themselves jealous of their peers. Financially, does it make sense to take on this debt and add more as I go through residency? Moreover, if you specialize, that takes even more years, which means more debt. Is this a good investment? When will my net worth ever become positive? All these thoughts and concerns, if not managed appropriately prior to residency, can destroy individuals and more importantly, their families.

So here is some advice. During the last few months prior to residency, one must READ! As hard as it may sound, always refresh your memory. I made the mistake of taking the last six months of my fourth year as vacation. I was done in December and had gone to India for several weeks. It was a lot of fun, but I was so unprepared for that first day. I remember strolling in to the hospital at seven in the morning for internal medicine rounds, which is absolutely ridiculous when you have eight new patients to see. I was new to the hospital, new to the area, did not know where to meet my team that morning. So, after finding my way to the team room, I was met by my senior resident who immediately was disgusted and knew it was going to be a long month. I ran around the hospital learning these patients as fast as I could. Time was my nemesis. My coat was holding me down as it was full of stupid handbooks that I never had time to sit and open. Now that I think about it, why do we carry these enormous handbooks, as if we think that the information will be somehow absorbed into our brain by some magical process of osmosis if we carry them; I guess, it gives us a sense of security knowing that the answer lies in our pockets.

My attending looked at my sweaty face and simply laughed. She knew I had come in late that morning and that there was no way I had seen all my patients in preparation for morning rounds. I was embarrassed and exhausted. So, note to self, arrive early and give yourself a lot of time, especially the first few weeks. It allows you to learn the system and begin the process of establishing a way of processing information. Next, you have to figure out a system where you can write down notes and have them accessible for rounds. Finally, for God sake, do not pack your lab coat with useless books!

One must develop a thick skin. The beauty of medical school rotations is that it helps us build a thick skin. You hear humiliating comments and get treated as useless members of a medical team early on in your rotations. So, by the time you are a resident, you have it down on what to do when an attending embarrasses you or other ancillary staff members treat you with disrespect.

However, I have noticed some residents have this belief that they know everything once they graduate medical school and actually end up disrespecting others. This is where education and awareness must take place. One must humble themselves first and foremost. No one can know everything and part of being human is to error. One must accept that. Moreover, humbleness facilitates a team atmosphere where no single member is felt to be dominating over the others. It is this simple virtue that will allow you to learn without being distracted by disturbing comments or disrespect that you may encounter. I believe that when you understand your own limitations as a human being, you allow yourself to forgive yourself and to learn from your mistakes. This is the most important lesson of all.

Take criticism as motivation. Sure, the competitive atmosphere can be quite stressful and each criticism can be taken as a loss. But, progress and self-improvement over time become more meaningful and will impress your staff. More importantly, remind yourself, you are not training to please your staff. You are training to become a better physician and gain the experience necessary to efficiently and effectively practice your business of medicine. So, criticism should be taken as motivation to improve your practice, adapt to change, and solidify your knowledge. The reality is that there are several physicians who act as if they know everything, however, recognize that every single person has strengths and weaknesses. Although one may have an enormous knowledge base and can recall the most minute detail of medical pathologies, the practice of medicine is more than just vomiting facts. It is a business. So, work on your communication skills, your bedside manner, coordinating care, and truly "managing" patient care. Understand the economics of the patient care you are delivering. In any competitive marketplace people will criticize you to slow your progress or gain insight into your business practice only to use it themselves to improve their business. You must be careful.

Moreover, in the day and age of advanced technology and social media, recognize that your early days of residency can pay dividends when you start your practice. Patients begin to learn who you are, experience your bedside manner, and will talk about you once you leave the room. Have business cards handy to provide to your patients because undoubtedly the patient with the laptop is not shopping online, instead they are staring at a blinking cursor waiting to comment on their experience with you.

Word of mouth is the best marketing vehicle for any business. Once you gain trust of your consumers, your business will be welcomed and progress is inevitable. In the same way, any physician that is trusted by their patients, will inevitably have a thriving practice. The question may become, what about those physicians who are not in solo practice and are instead employed by the hospital. Can this still play a major role? The answer is yes. Many of your colleagues are monitoring and observing how patients respond to your care.

More importantly, patients and their families are not shy to let staff know of their experience with their residents. Positive feedback will put big smiles on the staff members because they obviously will look good, but administration will smile as well. Patient satisfaction is a significant component in the business of health care delivery. Thus, from the moment you step into the hospital on the first day of residency, recognize that you are starting with an empty canvas. Only you can paint that canvas any way you want. In the end, everyone will be able to see what you have done with that canvas. Once it is done, it is extremely difficult to change the colors or the look of the overall canvas. Invest the time to make it as unique, colorful, and appealing as you can. We all get one canvas, no more.

Finally, each and every future resident must develop mental toughness and passion for what they do. It is these two characteristics that are the foundations for a successful medical career. The sad thing is that these two characteristics cannot be taught nor given to you. It is something you have to develop yourself. Fact of the matter is, just like Cooperate America, every physician is for him/herself. It's a business and every physician is looking out for themselves. So, throw away your belief that somebody will step in and help you when you are completely exhausted or beating yourself up for not doing the best job; instead, others who are competing for similar positions will be rejoicing behind your back. Hospitals are more concerned with the bottom line than ever before.

Physicians are their vehicles to market the great care their hospitals provide. If the hospital is not getting production, they can simply replace their physicians like any other business. Moreover, more physicians are becoming employees instead of small business owners with their own clinics given the unfortunate rising costs of owning a private practice. This feeds the bellies of Corporate America as hospitals are flooded with more applications and are allowed to impose more control over their physicians. Where else will they go?

I learned this the hard way. In the first several months of residency, there were no limitations to how much physical labor I did. For example, I would stay at the hospital into the late hours checking and double checking my work. My thought was that the more I did, the more I would learn, and the more my staff would appreciate my diligence. Some residents I came to know would sleep at the hospital daily! Usually these were the residents that were single.

I soon found myself immersed in the details, which only confused the overall clinical picture. I wanted everything to make sense like a nice story with a beginning and an end. This compromised my ability to see the big picture. I could not handle not knowing why certain things were happening to patients. Why is it that a normal human being without any risk factors, who exercises and eats right, have a heart attack? Moreover, how can this loving father of four children with no significant history get stage four colon cancer at the age of 55? It did not make sense.

The emotions of each case, the family meetings, the late night conversations with the patients, were beginning to consume me. How can one separate their emotions from each case? How is it that a physician can go from one room where they discuss terminal illness then enter the room right next to it and be joyful with the progress another patient makes? Moreover, how does this rollercoaster of emotions not be appreciated nor recognized by the general public?

Each case adds to ones overall perspective on life. You meet all kinds of people: various races, personal backgrounds, socioeconomic backgrounds, and of course personalities. What is even more fascinating is the variety of perspectives each individual has on the same diagnosis. For example, a diagnosis of cancer to some is like a death sentence. To others, it is taken as "we all have to go some time!" The human element is what is so special in the practice of medicine. There is no other business in this world where the service you provide will have lasting impact on the consumer. The words you say the minute you open your mouth are heard with the most eager set of ears.

Your audience is a room full of family members whose lives will also be affected the minute you start revealing the diagnosis and the treatment plan. It truly is a remarkable position to be in and one that must be taken with the utmost compassion.

As a young resident, you barely have time to reflect on yourself. Each case is introduced to you like a factory where you solve one and are presented immediately with another; usually more complicated than the previous with a whole new set of personalities. The social dynamics of each case also become a critical element of each case. The stories of elder abuse, domestic abuse, drugs, poverty, and violence complicate each case even further. This is why it is critical a physician observes their patients while obtaining the history. It is quite amazing the dynamics one can note in an exam room when the patient starts to tell their story. Are they maintaining eye contact? Why or why not? Is it a culture issue or are they not telling the truth? Why is that certain person in the room continuously interrupting our conversation? Why are their words not making sense? Why is this elderly woman's clothes so dirty and she smells like she has not showered? Why are the family members not here for this 75 year old woman who looks so malnourished?

It is more than listening during each physician interaction; its observation and taking mental notes of the social dynamics of each case. Imagine doing this almost thirty times a day for the rest of your life! When you are a young resident, this complexity of patient care is not appreciated and not taken seriously. Are we ever taught how to manage our emotions? Are we ever taught how to stay compassionate in a society where people try to manipulate the system to get free care or narcotics only to abuse them later?

As we progress in our residency training, we start to put our experiences into perspective. We formulate our style of patient care. Moreover, I am willing to bet that these experiences most definitely shape our view on life. A lot of our personal concerns become obsolete when we compare ourselves to those who are more unfortunate.

By December of my first year of residency, I hit rock bottom. It was too much. The hours, the lack of time spent with my wife, and the monotonous routine of each day was killing me. I thought about quitting almost every day for the next couple of months. I was tired of being "just a resident", being a reporter of the evening events when people can look for themselves, and getting the look from people that says, "well, he's just an intern." I was sick of it. I was annoyed by people who pretended they knew everything and walked around the hospital like they were seasoned physicians when in reality they were just second year residents. My thoughts poured into my attitude and life simply was not enjoyable. This was the breaking point. I think this is the crossroads every resident reaches around this time whether they admit it or not. The question remains, is this the best way of training our residents?

There came a point where I sat one night in the stairwell and stared at the empty wall in front of me. I was exhausted. Silence can be a good thing at times. Especially in a hospital where pagers, beeps from machines, and the random chatter of the wards consume ones mind and prohibit any rational thought outside of the task at hand. I simply was exhausted. I felt my years were passing by without much enjoyment. Was this truly worth it? I kept thinking of the large amount of student loans I had accumulated. How will I ever pay this back? How stupid is it that we put more stress on our young physicians by allowing colleges and medical colleges to charge monstrous tuitions? Sure there is student aide, but they are making even more money on that! The banks make three to five times the loan amount with interest! It is so absurd! How can we allow this to happen? Why not get another graduate degree for a quarter to half the cost and make just as much money?

But, I couldn't do that. I love medicine and the practice of medicine is more than just a job. It is a way of life, a privilege, an honor to be in a position to make a difference each and every day. Sure it was hard, but there is no other business in the world where I can go to sleep at night and be pleased with the difference I had made in someone's life. Sure there will be people who may not appreciate the time and energy you put into a treatment plan. But some day, they will realize that your hard work just improved their quality of life. More importantly, I knew I had to make changes in our health care system. I was just a resident at the time. But I had to complete my training, become the best physician I can be to help those who are left behind. This is why most of us physicians believe that the practice of medicine is a calling, where we feel the need to change this inefficient and broken system. I had to fight this green monster tattooed with dollar bills that was bringing corporate principles and capitalist influences into our hospitals and health systems; destroying the fundamental practice of medicine.

It is at this very moment that I made a decision and never looked back.

I wanted to do medicine and enjoyed every minute of it. I loved discussing pathologies with patients, and especially their families. I loved teaching and realized that night I was officially in the business. I am not a student. My actions now will establish a foundation for my future practice. This single thought energized me. I did not have to be like other residents, do things their way, talk their way, or behave their way for it to be the right way. The practice of medicine does not have a single best method. It's a business. So, I had to develop a method of delivering care that increased my effectiveness, marketability, and most importantly improve the quality of life. The beauty of being a physician is that while treating your patients, you are marketing yourself in the cheapest way possible. I also realized that as long as you did the right thing in each case and did your absolute best, no one can question your effort or decisions you had made. Moreover, knowledge is power. The more prepared I was, the more confidence I gained. I transitioned from working each day to get approval from others to working for myself and my family. The reality is, no attending, program director, or administrator truly cares about your career or the amount of money you make. Each only cares about their immediate concerns which are performance measures; board pass rates and production. Each attending will forget you by the time you complete your residency. So stop trying to impress them or even care what they think about you, because at the end of the day you should learn and work hard for yourself; no one else.

When you realize this, the possibilities are endless. Passion and mental toughness will help you plow through any barriers people may present in front of you and reach your goals. At the end of the day, it is your friends and family that matter most.

CHAPTER 16

Advice for the Family of the Young Resident

It is quite difficult to be the loved one whose spouse is a medical resident. Most of us do not realize nor appreciate the sacrifice they make. Today, there are support groups on the web and also at local hospitals that facilitate what we are about to discuss. It becomes evident from the previous chapters the rigors of medical residency can place substantial emotional, psychological, and financial burden on the resident and their support system. So, the question remains, how do we manage this entire burden?

The most important step is acceptance. This is where the family and loved ones must recognize that the medical resident will not be available for every gathering or family event. Time is not managed by them, but their program and have little control over when exactly they can get days off. There is some discussion when making the schedule, but for the most part, it is difficult to get every request. So, we must accept that time will be difficult to manage. We have to be flexible with our plans and arrangements.

Personally, it was a process for this to occur. It is easily said than done. As the months pass, it becomes clear of how much time we really have for other things. The fact of the matter is that the medical resident will be at the hospital usually from six in the morning to around five or six at night. Once they get home, one must read, prepare presentations for morning rounds, or research as part of working towards obtaining a fellowship or furthering their career. The crazy thing is that we do this around the clock! Even on weekends and holidays! When you are on a medicine, cardiology, or a nephrology service, there needs to be weekend coverage as well. So, it is very difficult to make plans.

One solution to this is to talk early on about future gatherings or family events. We are talking months in advance to facilitate the medical resident in making their requests. In terms of the week, spouses must stay proactive and discuss events weeks prior to the desired time. This will facilitate the possibility of accomplishing that arrangement. It sounds ridiculous, but emails or sending emails as appointments where you can accept and it will put it on your calendar, really works! My wife started doing this where she would send me emails as appointments and I simply had to accept them; automatically reserving that time slot in my calendar. Post It, white boards, and notes all help improve the communication when it comes to time management.

When it comes to family occasions, gatherings have to be prioritized. If you are single, then this may not be as big of an issue. But, when you are married, you have not only your side of the family, but you also have to consider your in-laws. Thus, married couples must communicate and compromise on which occasions are most important. Reality is, you cannot expect to be at every birthday, barbecue, or even weddings. This is the ultimate sacrifice each spouse has to make and be prepared to make. At the same time, residents must take note of all the sacrifices their spouse makes, because at some point you should return the favor.

The second is that the support system, mainly we are talking about the spouse, must make an effort to step up and help out with several things. This can range from the house bills to even applications related to medical residency or fellowship. It is amazing how fast time passes and deadlines, if left for the resident to remember, will be missed. We had a folder full of papers and my wife did a fantastic job of making calls, paying bills, and facilitating my applications during that busy time. Three years of residency seem long on paper, but they pass quite quickly. The family unit should have clear communication and understanding of their overall goals. Both husband and wife should work towards making clear plans for reaching those goals to sustain the family. This is tough. It requires patience and diligence to set a few goals every few months. These goals can be time spent together, financial goals in terms of loan interest payments or savings, or educational goals. Nonetheless, these must be discussed so that there is clear communication from the start. When the time does starts to pass quickly, there is an understanding among one another; thus, eliminating or reducing the frustration that comes innately with any residency.

Each goal should be reassessed. Financial goals for example should be assessed from a monthly to quarterly basis. We assessed our finances each month and used excel to help analyze our finances. It is cheap and easy way to create a chart to see where your dollars are spent. It does take time to input the data, but that single investment will help future budget planning and is vital for debt reduction in forecasting future financial decisions. Even pen and paper work. In fact, I started off this way and made charts with one side listed all the credit cards and another listed my student loans. It helps to see on a monthly basis how you are spending towards reducing this debt. It gives you some precision in your finances and helps you make more informed decisions. There are software programs out there like Microsoft Money and Quicken. My experience with these programs is that they simply do not categorize your expenses accurately. You end up fixing the data more than analyzing and formulating information from that data.

Pay attention to amortization schedules and pay a little more towards reducing your debt if you can. Although student loans offer forbearance or even deferment for only a fixed amount of time, it is best to pay the interest or whatever you are able to pay towards the principal during your residency years. There is a fixed amount you can claim on you taxes when payments are paid towards your student loan, so researching the current rates is important.

In reflection of my own experience, communication was learned over time and unfortunately was not my greatest asset from the start. This may actually sound surprising as I minored in communication studies and have always been an advocate for improving communication when it comes to system processes. But, I think that it is true for most of us that when it comes to our own life, we tend to forget what we preach at times. There are several things in our lives we wish we did things differently. Well, this is one of those things. It is the main goal of this book to share lessons like this for future residents, so that hopefully they can be better prepared. The problem is, we do not appreciate the complexity and the difficulty of what we are about to face at the beginning of residency. By the time we realize the road has become rocky and the terrain starts to get rough. We look back and realize it may be too late to re-trace your steps. The truth of the matter is that it is never too late to reflect, reassess, and redirect yourself when you recognize it. The most important component is that you realize that the course has been diverted; this realization can be from the spouse or the resident or both. The next step is to accept it, not ignore it or hope over time things will get better without addressing the issues. As hard as it may be, one must sit down, gather their thoughts, maximize their patience, and start to brainstorm solutions to each challenge.

Words are powerful, irreversible, and can do more damage that one may think. It is critical we control our emotions that churn within us, because once those emotions are translated to words, there is no turning back. The receiver starts to take that message and process it. And no matter how much you try to retrieve the message, the bottom line is, it has already been processed and certain emotions and thoughts have already been initiated by the other person. So, the best way to eliminate words that unfortunately have been said is to accept the fact that it will take time and action to show the contrary. One must stay patient and focused on their goal of eliminating these unfortunate messages. After some time, there needs to be some reminders like, "I'm sorry I said this, but I am trying to show you that I didn't mean it. I know it will take time." I think that as long as two people love each other, innately they will forgive each other. It just takes time. Moreover, I think that deep down in their hearts, they probably have already forgiven you because they love you. So, this should bring confidence and worth towards implementing actions towards eliminating unfortunate communications from the past. Time seems to lag, but be confident that over time, the future is filled with happiness.

Thus, the team model exists even in the home. The resident and their respective families must work together to obtain their goals. Patience, mental toughness, and organization will bring success to any family. Like any team, one must surround themselves with the right players.

So, the resident obviously must focus on stabilizing and leading his/her family, but also must be quick to seek resources when help is needed. Let's dissect this further.

Earlier in our discussion we discussed the financial burdens medical education places on families. Therefore, it follows that one must get a trustworthy accountant and financial planner to help reduce this burden. Reality is that medical residents are not trained regarding finances and how to manage their debt. Banks are quick to throw educational loans at you with nice interest rates, because they know you will have the income to pay in the future resulting in a huge profit for them; little do they care about how much burden it puts on you and your family. In addition, even though the salary of a resident is small, it is very important to build savings. There should be two purposes for savings.

One is for the long term. If your spouse works, you should consider a Roth IRA if you meet those requirements. A Roth IRA will allow you to contribute to this retirement fund with a tax benefit. Second, you should have an emergency fund, because we all know things happen in life despite our careful planning. This will limit your immediate cash flow, but for the first several months, I would be aggressive and save. You can certainly dine at home more, limit the movies, and entertainment for some time. Truth is, no one cares about your money more than you and your family, so you must manage it. Financial planners are great for ideas and help with organizing a plan for attacking your loans. But please be careful.

Anybody can call themselves a financial planner. Even some of these salesmen for large financial firms will call themselves financial planners. Their goal is to simply sell you financial products and squeeze their way into knowing your finances so they can convince you that you can afford their financial products. Moreover, you must read and be informed before you sign on the dotted line for any financial product. Everybody knows you will make decent income when you graduate so they would like to start building relationships now for long term gains. Do not trust people easily. They will find ways into your pockets and the consensus in the financial world is that physicians are easy prey since they have deep pockets with little financial knowledge. So, please be careful and do not let greed overcome your personal and family vision. Patience, research, and careful analysis will bring financial success. It is easy to seek the quick dollar, but the reality is that there is no such thing as a "quick buck." Sure, people get lucky with markets and investments, but you must learn to diversify your portfolio, spread the risk, and learn prior to making investments. Careful planning is essential. Never lose sight of your vision and your family; because your mistakes may impact more than just you.

If you can, pay interest on your loans as this will help with tax savings. This is where an accountant will help. Donate old clothes! Give donations, seek tax saving financial vehicles, and keep a track of your own spending to assess your monthly expenditures so you know where to make some cuts. Investing in a good accountant will pay for itself. If your taxes are relatively simple, TurboTax is pretty good too. Finally, I would recommend investing in life insurance and disability while you are young. It is cheaper and quite honestly, it protects your family and provides them with resources should something happen to you. Life insurance and disability insurance are important. However, one must read prior to buying these insurances. There is much to learn and even after reading, I guarantee you will have questions. This is where an unbiased financial planner can help you. Again, be aware of financial planners that simply call themselves financial planners and are not certified. Many insurance companies have sales agents that call themselves financial planners; when in reality, they are simply selling their products. There are several books on investing, finding the right financial planner, and taxes. Pick up any one of these books and read. The "Dummy's" version is always a good place to start.

So, it becomes clear that the resident and the family are a unit who must work together and surround themselves with players that will help them meet their goals. Financial resources are very important as you progress in residency. It will prepare you for managing your debt, give you confidence in managing your money, and finally, allow you to make informed financial decisions when out of residency. Never hesitate to ask questions and to admit that you do not know about certain topics. We tend to shy away from topics we are least acquainted with or have less knowledge. We like to read about things we already know or have some familiarity. This is what gets young physicians in trouble. Our brains are not trained to seek other information or even have a taste for financial knowledge. How many times have we heard physicians say "well, I am not doing this for the money and I don't care. I just want to take care of patients." Reality is, you have to care. No medical practice can exist without financial funding and the physician themselves cannot exist without financial security. The expenses at some point will overcome revenue if not managed appropriately. So the question remains, how can we better prepare these young physicians for the real-world?

CHAPTER 17

Advice for Residency Programs

Residency programs have done tremendous work towards reducing duty hours and increasing the volume of resident's they accept into the program. The question remains, is this enough? By limiting duty hours, are we limiting their learning experience? Can we trust that the time these residents have available with the new duty hours will be spent reading? All these are difficult questions to answer in this short section. However, the answer must start with the resident taking on the responsibility themselves.

If the resident is determined to be the best, the most informed, and work hard during these training years, then the answer is no. We are not limiting their learning experience, nor will we be hesitant whether or not they will use that free time wisely. It is the resident who must seek knowledge. It is the goal of this book to teach young physicians the importance of seeking knowledge to be more informed physicians. No one will sit and tell you exactly what you need to do or learn in order to be the best physician possible. The unfortunate truth is that just as any other business, competition is fierce among physicians. Residents may not tell you, but knowledge is not shared as freely as one would think, like in any competitive setting.

So, to provide more succinct advice to residents, you must read about the various pathologies that you encounter on the wards, but at the same time, one must seek knowledge regarding health systems and public policy. The sad reality is, we have very little to none lectures regarding health systems or health law. There is not much motivation and emphasis placed on the importance of these topics by our teaching staff. In the mist of seeing 15-18 patients, it is difficult to do teaching that is inclusive of pathology and health systems.

Therefore, it is imperative that the resident spend their free time learning about the social and systemic issues regarding each case. Moreover, simply paying attention to public health policy will raise awareness. Attending conferences and participating in various committee activities will introduce residents to health policy, law, finance, and management. But again, it is the responsibility of the resident to seek opportunities where they can obtain this knowledge and use their free time to attend conferences and meeting where public policy and health systems are discussed.

The resident council offers such an environment. This council is composed of residents from across multiple specialties to address resident issues. The leadership of the resident council is allowed to participate with the Graduate Medical Education meeting where all the program directors meet and discuss various topics. This experience can provide numerous benefits including gaining an understanding of health systems and start building leadership skills outside the direct delivery of patient care.

Other examples of committee involvement include infection control, quality and safety, and information technology. Involving residents as part of these committees has benefits that cannot be taught in lectures or grand rounds. In addition, it will encourage the resident to manage time effectively and master the art of multi-tasking. Medical staff and administration should provide encouragement and facilitate an environment where the resident is empowered to make some decisions and present their ideas. It should be more than simple attendance to meetings. It requires full participation from administration and medical staff to facilitate this experience. Nonetheless, all students need teachers, mentors, and resources to facilitate such knowledge to be obtained.

Thus, residency programs can help change the quality of our young physicians and allow them to improve themselves by providing a culture of learning. This culture of learning must entail opportunities for mistakes, empower all of its staff members, be flexible such that new ideas may allow changes to improve system processes, allow for communication to flow freely in every direction, involve the most enthusiastic teaching physicians to maintain that energy on the wards daily, and finally allow resident leadership opportunities. This culture must be shared from administration to the nurses and all the way down to the volunteers in the hospital. Organizational culture is critical to its overall success. Therefore, establishing this culture is critical. How can residency programs do that?

First and foremost, there must be buy in from administration. This has to be a system wide process. You cannot have a residency program subculture submerged in a dominant system culture where the program cannot thrive. It makes no sense and unfortunately we see this happening today. Administration must realize that residency programs are critical to their overall existence and can certainly add significant value to their organization if managed appropriately. What we are talking about here is good for any hospital. So, this should not be hard. The culture of learning should be implemented in every hospital.

A residency program can help administration recognize the benefits of establishing a culture of learning by doing it themselves. Besides, residents see the most patients anyway and interact with ancillary staff more than administration. Thus, residency programs can encourage this and be quite effective in establishing this culture system wide with some simple maneuvers.

The first step is to teach their residents and empower them to be leaders. This means teaching residents to communicate effectively with ancillary staff. Leading rounds and be part of the daily rounds; more than simply regurgitating overnight events. They should be allowed to run rounds with the staff physician at their side evaluating their progress. There should be constant feedback between staff and their residents in how to coordinate, manage, and lead treatment teams (the nurse, the social work, case manager, pharmacist, patient and their families). The residents should be taught to be patient and work on building links with nurses to form a team approach to patient care. In addition, bridges should be made where all medical staff members involved in a case are constantly working together towards providing care for a single patient.

Nurses should be empowered to make some decisions and work with residents and their staff in managing patient care. Protocols are great for assuring standard of care is implemented, but the protocol should not be the only guidance in patient care. We must lift the red tape, the ridiculous amount of protocols that limit a nurse from being a true nurse. Today, they are inundated with so many check lists that they do not have time to think about the pathophysiology of what is actually occurring. For example, they have to call physicians about any abnormal vitals. So it is not uncommon to get a call about a blood pressure of 160/80. That is all that is communicated to the physician. Then the annoying question is follows, "what do you want me to do about it?"

Well, what are the other vitals? Is the patient in pain? What are the heart sounds like and what is the heart rate? Is the patient in distress? Any lab changes this morning? Is this different from previous blood pressure measurements overnight? So, you see, all these questions must be answered by the nurse before making that call. Therefore, it allows for a conversation to occur, instead of a single question/answer interaction. We need to move away from practicing medicine in a reactive way. More conversations and analysis must occur on the wards.

Nurses are in demand today more than ever. Hospitals are putting more beds while fewer nurses are hired to care for those new beds. It does not make sense. So as the patient to nurse ratios get worse, meaning one nurse is handling more patients, it threatens patient safety. Moreover, the entire treatment team will suffer because each nurse is not involved with their patient as they should be. Again, if nurses have fewer patients to take care of, they will be able to know why the patient came to the hospital, be able to remember their medical history better, and will be an active member of the rounding team when it comes to making some decisions.

Residents must be taught to be patient and become teachers on the wards. They must lead by example by helping nurses and the rest of the treatment team feel part of the team. They must be able to empower each member with the ability to take part in making decisions towards patient care. Again, everyone may have an opinion, thus it is imperative a respectful conversation take place at the bedside. When residents start to do this across specialties and system wide, hospital staff will take note and the culture of leaning will slowly be established.

Part of organizational culture is vision and mission statements, artifacts around the hospital, the communications that take place around the hospital, and the overall attitude of its staff. As residents start to teach on the wards, interact with ancillary staff in ways to establish this culture, they can further implement the principles of this culture when they take leadership positions in various hospital committees.

When I was president of our resident council, it was quite difficult at first. This council was brand new and we invited several residents from various specialties to be part of the council. In addition, it is quite intimidating to be shoulder to shoulder with some of the program directors when attending the Graduate Medical Education (GME) meetings. I was also called to make updates during these meetings, which was nerve wrecking at first, but became a great opportunity to voice resident concerns to program directors. I found that program directors truly care about their residents and want each of them to be the best. Thus, the environment in that board room was inviting such that I was able to find comfort in sharing our recent progress at council meetings. We had an administrator that was our mentor and guided us in how to run efficient meetings. The resident council is a huge success and residents love having a voice at the table. So, it is not hard to do this as long as the organization will accept change and seek to establish a culture of learning.

CHAPTER 18

Advice for Residency Program Directors

And

The Medical Community

Program directors across the country must recognize this need and find solutions to this growing problem. There is a huge gap between physicians and lack of business knowledge. Young physicians need guidance and encouragement to pick up the newspaper and understand present-day issues. In the mist of this health care debate, how many young physicians truly understand what is happening and what are the key issues that are being debated? Do they understand how it will affect their practice? It seems that no one talks about these issues during residency or medical school as if it will never affect our future practice. Or is it that we shy away from this topic, because understanding it would require us to learn terminology and concepts that we have no knowledge of prior to even scratching the surface of the issues at hand?

It is a real problem. I remember being asked as a resident what I thought about the health care debate. I did not have a well formed answer. This experience left me embarrassed, so much so that I sought to go to a meeting where they discussed the active issues at a nearby conference center. It is quite sad to see these young graduates who have no idea the challenges of the real world, and once they enter it, they remain dazed and confused. More importantly, it is extremely sad to see graduates have no idea how to handle their finances.

No physician will become rich by simply being a physician. There are enough barriers from taxes, lack of stock options, to subpar retirement plans offered by hospitals. You see, in business, there is an unlimited amount of earning potential. Private office practices offer this illusion, but in reality, the reimbursement rates will prevent this from ever happening; thus, the flux of internists towards hospitalist medicine or establishment of large multi-group practices. It is no wonder you see physicians on commercials endorsing pathetic products or participating with pharmaceutical industries by giving lectures about medications they may not completely support. Where are the incentives to promote more production or prevent physicians from becoming employees of hospitals? Part of the small business economy includes small office practices. Imagine the job creation potential if these outpatient practices are supported by improving reimbursement rates, providing incentives for the establishment of solo practitioners and preventative medicine.

Patients are the ones who suffer from this shortage of primary care physicians. There are numerous stories across the country where patients are left looking for another primary care physician because their primary care physician left their practice to become hospitalists or some fellowship to become a specialist. Small office practices offer a personal touch to medicine and allow the possibility for patients and physicians to build lasting relationships. It is through these partnerships that the health of a community can achieve lasting improvements. Imagine the credibility, trust, and buy-in a community physician can have on local health issues. Thus, small practices should be supported such that public local projects can be sought to improve their communities. This simple concept will improve job satisfaction from the primary care perspective and the community will benefit from the leadership of a local physician. Thus, it is imperative that we incentivize the development of local public health programs.

From an educator's perspective, we must recognize this need for the production of primary care physicians. We must work towards encouraging our young physicians to embrace the leadership of being a primary care provider. Students should be able to appreciate and recognize the benefits of managing an outpatient primary care practice.

Thus, if the system allows for the growth of private practice, outpatient practice, and educators mobilize to encourage the development of primary care providers, then the growth of primary care is inevitable.

In light of the whole health care debate and rising health care costs, the problem seems simple. The incentives are not in line to motivate young physicians to choose primary care as a profession when compared to the salaries and earning potential of specialists. Moreover, I wonder if more young physicians would choose primary care if they understood the business of medicine and the potential opportunities that may be overlooked simply because they lack business training.

The worsening economy has also been in the headlines. What if we trained our physicians to be entrepreneurs or equipped them with tools to establish a successful business? A major component of our economy is entrepreneurship, which gives rise to small businesses – ultimately increasing jobs. Physicians find themselves seeking leadership positions and administrators are recognizing the importance of physician leadership. However, the challenges arise when physicians find themselves in leadership positions and are ineffective simply because of their inability to communicate with a team or make financial decisions. Would it not be beneficial to health care organizations to hire physicians with some basic management skills to leadership positions? Therefore, it is common sense to invest in our young physicians to improve our global economy.

Young physicians should be exposed to management, finance, and communication studies early in their careers. I would argue, this must start in pre-med classes. Have students interact with the business school. I remember the pre-med crowd was separated from the business school. It was as if we had no connection or no idea what the other side of campus had to offer. Courses allow assimilation and encourage discussions where scientific minds are forced to utilize another part of their brain. When I was taking my courses towards my MHA, each night class was like discovering a new skill I never thought I had. There is an explosion of new ideas, thought processes, and analysis that you would never have to use in medical school or basic sciences. Much of medicine is memorizing disease processes and making analytical decisions based on probability and research. Finance and management require analysis that is much different than medical decision-making.

In medical school, students need to be taught public policy, management, and communication studies early in their training. The first year should include some of these courses. Management and human resources training is critical by their second year as this is the year just before their rotations. Students need to learn the importance of recognizing system process, motivating employees, working as a team leader, the importance of collaboration, and how to recruit and retain staff. This is just the surface of the skills they would obtain from taking these courses. Marketing is also important to understand and having the ability create a strategic plan is a tremendous asset for any leader. During rotations, medical students get busy on the wards, but what about having on-line courses available? Certainly, medical students are done by 5pm and can attend these courses on-line. Much of learning has to be done by the individual and these on-line courses make discussions feasible, especially now with so many options to gather people together via the web. There are several options to implement this education and students should demand it.

In residency, life gets only busier and faster. This is why it is critical that education and training start early in this whole process. Students and residents always ask the question, "well, why do I need to know this right now?" or they will say, "I can learn this later." The fact is that once you graduate it, life gets even busier. New job, new hospital, family pressures, and of course your loans will go into repayment, so guess who will be working the extra shifts to make some extra cash to pay these loans?

Therefore, we need to increase the awareness of our medical residents about the importance of taking advantage of their training years and optimize their education. There will never be more time. More importantly, it will delay the success and opportunities you would have if you had the financial training earlier. Trust me, you would be more confident, take on leadership roles with ease, and make some solid financial decisions once out of residency. I had so many of my fellow residents that would say they will learn as they progress in their medical career, but the reality is that it takes a lot of time. Think about it. If you had no financial background, how can you make sense of financial statements or the financial vision of your hospital? How can you propose a reasonable budget analysis or stakeholder analysis prior to proposing a policy change? If you go into solo practice, how do you even begin to manage your finances or if you hire someone to manage for you, will you be able to check their work? How can you trust others with your money?

These are critical questions that must be recognized and answered by every resident. Only then will they realize the importance of this discussion. You see, people don't care if these young physicians are trained or equipped with financial knowledge. In fact, the word on the street is to seek young physicians to get a hold of their pocketbooks, because they simply have no idea how to manage it. In the real world, people will approach physicians with extravagant business plans and ideas and will request some investment. The novice physicians will usually invest without a thorough research. Sure, they will surf the web for articles and ask their colleagues, but this does not equal the research and analysis one would make with some business training. So, young physicians are walking around with a sign on their head saying "come and talk to me, I have no idea what to do with my money!"

Worse yet is the spending binge these physicians do once they graduate. The new cars and houses get them into financial trouble. First thing is first. Focus on debt reduction. Student loans are not assets. Focus on the loan with the highest interest rate and get aggressive. Create a plan for each loan and work towards meeting those goals strictly. Cut the entertainment expenses if you have to because this investment will create opportunities for the future. Start saving early and compromise at nothing. Start your retirement fund early as well. Seek knowledge of further investments to allow your money to grow. If you are saving for a house, it will take time to build enough cash for a down payment while saving and paying down debt. You have to include some surplus cash for repairs, moving in, and other starting up expenses. That is ok. No one expects you to roll around in a jaguar the minute you graduate. Besides, practicing medicine itself will not make you filthy rich, you must get over that concept.

Saving, paying debt, tax saving, and reducing expenses must start in residency. This concept must be taught and encouraged in residency. Programs can offer morning report lectures, grand rounds lectures, and financial counseling that is required for each resident. It makes no sense to provide financial counseling as an elective or as needed. No resident will stop what they are doing; go to the other side of the hospital, only to see a financial counselor who may spend some thirty minutes with a tired resident who constantly reminds himself "I could have been sleeping right now."

Many businesses prey on the weaknesses of our young physicians. It is the ugly truth of a capitalistic society – every man for himself. No one will come to your aide if your financial reserves become empty. Instead, people will be interested in the story of the cycle of financial losses more than helping you find solutions and guide you back on track. Thus, the focus should be on prevention. In a day where media infiltrates our commercials, television shows, and articles regarding the rich and the famous, people around the world are becoming thirsty for that quick way to become those people. It is a false reality that the media creates, negating the other problems or issues that may surround these "rich and famous" people.

What makes matters worse is that we have young physicians who are even younger than ever before. People are going to the Caribbean's or other countries to accelerate the time it takes to become a physician. Here in the United States, we offer six to eight year accelerated programs to draw some of the brightest students towards skipping the college experience from high school and fast tracking them right into medical school. I see a lot of concerns regarding this path. Of course, every student is different, but we must admit those early years after high school are full of poor decisions and lack of responsibility. I have seen graduates from the Carribean or other countries come to America and struggle to pass their boards. The next several months to years of their career after graduating from foreign medical schools are consumed with passing these board exams. Sure, the boards will ask a few questions regarding health law or health care, which is usually memorized couple of days prior to the exam. But, we must ask what about the comprehension of our health system? What about understanding what managed care is or how Medicare and Medicade actually came to be in our health system? Outside of the basics, few understand the reimbursement system or even the market trends regarding the future of medical practice. Forget about practice management. If one does not understand the management skills of a business, nor do they understand the financial system and reimbursement rates, how will they understand how to manage their clinic? The usual answer is, "I'll learn in residency." Yeah, right.

So, how is it that we expect these medical students who graduate from these accelerated/foreign programs to find the time to learn about management, finance, or communication? Moreover, will they have the maturity to handle their finances once they graduate from these accelerated programs and enter residency? Even more concerning is, will they have the maturity and responsibility of handling their finances once they become part of the medical staff?

This is why it is critical that medical schools around the country mobilize towards strengthening the financial and business skills of our young physicians. There must be a safety net established in our residency programs to capture those students who are in accelerated programs, whether they be American graduates or foreign. At one spectrum, it helps the medical profession by training and establishing a more informed group of future physicians and on the other it will significantly help our global economy as these young physicians will be more willing to invest their dollars towards financial vehicles that support the global market.

The role of medical educators is changing. It is imperative that we recognize it and mobilize resources towards strengthening our programs. The curriculum in our pre-med courses must be reviewed. Courses in finance, management, and communication are important early in medical training. The medical schools need to continue this momentum with offerings of courses that involve human resources, marketing, accounting, and finance. Finally, residency must provide lectures and discussions to stimulate the growth of financial knowledge and comprehension of health systems and processes. It is only through these modifications and system-wide change that will improve our medical training; ultimately, improving the medical profession on a national and global level.

CHAPTER 19

As a Junior Staff Hospitalist

Since graduating from residency, working as a staff hospitalist is a very rewarding experience. All the skills you learn from college to residency are utilized to their most optimum potential. This reflection and discussion facilitate the establishment of a more personal style of practice. Every graduate and young staff physician should have an internal discussion that demands the optimal utilization of their knowledge and skills.

As a hospitalist, it becomes apparent quite quickly that leadership requires effective communication and management skills. Patient care is complex given not only the intricacies of their pathology but also the social issues that surround each patient. Coordination of care and management of each issue is a skill that comes with repetition and experience.

I find that patients and family members appreciate the complexity and the attention each patient demands when one sits down and explains each issue involved in delivering patient care. Arranging family meetings is a simple way to get families together to discuss the patients' case in great detail and allow questions to be addressed in the most efficient manner. From a physician perspective, this investment will help reduce the time it takes to explain things each day and may facilitate more efficient visits following the meeting. For the patient and their respective families, this will allow a time for questions to be answered and understand the issues at hand in a more relaxed environment. However, respect for one another and appreciation of the time that is given by both parties must be recognized and communicated to one another.

I am very blessed to be trained at a facility where it was quite visible how the internal medicine program was striving to improve their residency training. In the three years of my training, I have seen more push towards having residents on committees, building their leadership skills, while assuring their medical training is optimal.

At the same time, recent regulations for reducing duty hours for residents, the advent of PICC lines (central lines placed by specialty nurses via ultrasound), and limiting some autonomy for concerns of patient safety come with a double edge sword. Back in the seventies, residents had to draw their own blood as residents and help transport patients to the radiology suite if they wanted some type of imaging. Yeah, that was more like today's television show "House," where the students seem to do everything!

But in all seriousness, by drawing their own blood and assisting with transport, residents had to think twice before ordering blood tests or even imaging. The question of "do I really need this to make a diagnosis or help in my management?" were common on a daily basis. It is true that today's society is more litigious than before. We have to ask, how did we get away from asking the question? Is it solely because we practice more of defensive medicine? Or, is it because our physical exam is less effective or complete? Finally, or is it because as a society we expect and demand our physicians to order these blood tests and MRI's, etc to satisfy our need that everything was done to provide care for our loved one. The reality is that this approach is not cost effective and we all pay for it directly or indirectly whether we realize it or not.

My experience is that the American people want the best for their loved one, but it is very difficult to remind people of two things – death at some point is definite, and life cannot be enriched with money. No matter how much you spend, it does not equal quality of life. Our advanced technologies may prolong life, but we have to define quality of life for one another and communicate it to one another so that the entire family will know exactly how you define quality of life.

This requires patience and communication, which each physician must be able to do at minutes' notice, as life can surprise all of us at any given time. My master's degree in health administration has equipped me with these skills. Again, these courses build a foundation. They do not make me an expert. It is through the practice of the learned principles that expertise can be achieved. This is important to understand.

As a hospitalist, I also am involved with committees and recognize the importance of collaboration of resources to provide the most efficient and comprehensive patient care. Social workers, case managers, care coordinators, pharmacists, physical therapists, and speech therapists all are part of the treatment team. Let's not forget the nutritionist, nurses, various techs that are involved in each case. It is important to recognize and appreciate this dynamic model of patient care. Multiple specialists and professionals are involved in the delivery of patient care. However, the physician is the leader of this treatment team and must maintain the vision and overall goals as the patients clinical course evolves.

This is where managerial skills, marketing, and an understanding of finance helps. Length of stay, utilization of resources, and reducing cost are important for every hospitalist to keep in mind while creating and implementing a treatment plan for their patient population. Again, this is a dynamic process because it is influenced by the patient, family members, and the treatment team. Thus, all viewpoints and concerns must be taken under consideration before implementing and maintaining patient care. When one stands back and reflects on this process, it is quite impressive how fast we coordinate these treatment plans and treat patients in such short hospital days.

Finally, finance is the biggest issue that needs attention in our medical education. It is ridiculous how expensive it is to obtain an education in the United States. College tuition itself is on the rise. Sure, those financial offices offer student loans – like credit cards give you that false sense of security that you will be able to pay it later. But, with any interest rate, loans are simply money making operations that ultimately put the students at risk. It literally puts shackles around your heels and places the banks hand into your pockets to assure they have access to your income.

Student loans are simply a nightmare. Imagine, after fours of medical school, passing all boards, three years of residency, and finally finding a job only to find out that the original loan you had taken out has almost doubled over time because of interest. In addition, once in repayment, which is usually within six months of graduating, now you have to assure you have enough for basic life needs and your student loans. Some physicians may not care, but the longer you take to pay them off, the more the banks fill their stomachs with your money. This is where I felt there is a lack of preparation and the entire nation needs to make serious improvements regarding this matter. We must ask ourselves, is it financially worth it to go to medical school? Is it cost-effective? These are the same questions students are asking themselves prior to applying. Moreover, to make medicine more financially worthwhile, many will specialize. However, one must think about it twice before doing so as extra years in training mean more interest on your student loans. So, it must be a calculated decision. In addition, just because your salary may increase, you will enter a higher tax bracket, which means you pay higher taxes on your salary. There are no stock options, but you do get a 403b plan or some retirement package with a matching plan – do you think this will suffice for retirement? The answer is, quite honestly, nope.

This gives rise to the problems addressed in this book. Physicians will seek businesses, get loans to establish some business, or they will be suckered into some business scam only to find out later that they were played. It becomes apparent how our physicians are connected to our global market. The crash of our financial system cannot be blamed entirely on the banks for lending this money, but its business people, including physicians, asking for loans when they themselves may know they were unable to pay the debt.

Physicians must manage their debt before taking on more debt. Our medical education must support and provide incentives to encourage students to pursue a medical career. Medical students should not be talking about their student loans while trying to excel in their career. Residents should not have the burden of making ends meet for their family while working several hours a week during residency. You can reduce duty hours, but the reality is, medical training requires time at home which involves research and reading. Thus, no matter what the new regulations may be, time and financial management must be taught prior to entering residency. We must prepare and invest in our residents to improve the future of medicine.

The real world practice of medicine requires self-discipline and humbleness. As physicians, we tend to believe we are incredibly smart and have the ability to learn everything. This is obviously not true. Some of the worst financial decisions are made by physicians. We must be humble, seek knowledge, and recognize our weaknesses. Just as in medical practice, we must surround ourselves with proficient team members who can guide us towards better financial decisions.

The practice of medicine is far more than rounding on patients today. Physicians have enormous opportunities for leadership in hospitals and their communities. These are learning opportunities to improve and strengthen your skills. It is only through humbleness that a medical staff member is able to grow and make real changes in the medical profession. We must return to the ideology that being a physician is a privilege and an honor to treat the sick. As a nation, we must respect our caretakers and move towards improving our health care to maintain the health of the American people. A nation that has the inability to sustain the health of its people will inevitably become a weak nation.

Chapter 20

Final Thoughts...

The goal of this book was to increase the public awareness regarding our health care from the eyes and ears of the medical resident. In reflection of this book, one can see that the life of a medical resident is more than what Hollywood portrays on the big screen. Medical training is rigorous, demanding, challenging, and comprehensive. The problems and issues of our health care system must include our medical education. One may argue it is a result of our lack of comprehensive medical training. The incentives are not in the right place to promote small business and the spirit of entrepreneurship. In addition, debt is poorly managed, leading to frustrated physicians. The lack of business training of our young physicians facilitated poor financial decisions that ultimately affect our global economy.

The United States spends a large portion of its GDP on health care, so it follows then that we must evaluate our health system from all angles. This assessment must include not only the issue of insurance coverage, but also medical training as this directly or indirectly affects our global economy. The young physician is at an important time in history. There are enormous opportunities for change and to make significant difference in the delivery of patient care. The practice of medicine is larger than what it had been even five years ago. The advancements in technology and the break through research challenge all physicians. However, at the same time, the business of medicine is growing more complex. In a population of physicians who lack business training, the market growth is detrimental; leaving patients in difficult situations.

As young physicians in America, we must recognize this void and take it upon ourselves to learn and mobilize resources to improve the delivery of health care through advancing medical training. Most of us take part in academics after graduation and thus should make every effort to motivate our residents to learn the business practice of medicine. Just as the sciences are important for patient management, communication and coordination of patient care is just as important if not more. This concept must be recognized and taught.

Program directors, teachers, and mentors must find ways to "beef up" their curriculums with business training. There must be a discussion between pre-med training to residency training in creating possibilities and solutions towards maintaining a continuum of learning as each student progresses in their medical training. Colleges must find ways to increase the discussions and involvement between pre-med and business students. The campus should not be divided anymore. We must find ways to encourage pre-med students to enter our business classrooms.

The United States health care system has a lot of potential to be great. We are a nation that learns, adapts, and prides itself in spreading innovation throughout the world. All nations have strengths and weaknesses. We must look at our health care system from the ground up and look further than just the issue of insurance coverage. The troubles of our economy include our health care system. The root of our troubles comes down to education. The more informed we are, the better decisions we make, the more confident we are in managing our business, and ultimately the better care we provide for our patients.

The practice of medicine is in the business of providing a service. We certainly are doing a good job in creating complex systems and innovative ways of providing patient care, but those who are directly involved with patient care stay behind in participating with the business of providing comprehensive care.

As young physicians, we must not shy away from our weakness. Let's show the world that we are as strong as our pioneers who boast about making a diagnosis with only their stethoscope. We are a generation of physicians that will understand the influence and potential of our health care in the global market.

More importantly, our knowledge will lead to innovative solutions, ultimately reducing the cost of health care delivery by streamlining systems and processes, reducing unnecessary testing, and bringing back the respect primary care deserves. It is a time for reflection and a time to go back to the basics. We are human beings, not robots.

We live in a time where obesity is ingesting our country, not even leaving our children behind. Our health remains at significant jeopardy. As a society we must move towards healthy lifestyles, but the reality is we will need to seek health care at some point in our lives. It is a system that we cannot simply ignore. As a nation, we must invest in our health care system such that our physicians are able to focus on patient care without the financial burdens that are placed on them during their training years. We need physicians who understand the global market and invest their salaries towards improving the economy. We need them to have less debt so they can establish small businesses and be able to take on a business loan. Imagine the number of jobs that would open up if more physicians had private clinics or were more motivated to open group practices that provided educational and other services beyond the medical practice. This would open up more jobs, allow communities to perceive these clinics as their neighborhood education centers, and ultimately building stronger communities and a stronger nation.

Some physicians around the country have become creative and have biking events with patients and other activities to encourage physical fitness. This time would also allow the community to spend time with their physician outside the clinic. Why can we all not do this? Why do we not invest in primary care such that the amount of time spent in activities like this are more feasible across the country? These investments are more rewarding and more effective than a fifteen minute clinic visit. Relationships are built, motivation is born, and hopefully lasting lifestyle changes are made. This is what medicine should be about.

The practice of medicine must stop being a reactive practice and more towards prevention and education. As a society we must become more preventative and allow financial resources for people to afford a healthier way of life. Let's put an end to frivolous lawsuits, decrease the cost of medications, allow people the ability to seek preventative visits, and finally financially reward primary care physicians for seeing these patients; because the bottom line is that it is they who will save the country health care dollars and improve the health of our nation.

The time is now to better train our young physicians, get rid of the Hollywood stereotypes, and equip physicians with knowledge to become informed participants of our global economy.

www.ingramcontent.com/pod-product-compliance
Lightning Source LLC
Chambersburg PA
CBHW051325170526
45166CB00002B/684